50 *More* Ways to Abuse Your Voice

Another Singer's Guide to a Short Career

50 *More* Ways to Abuse Your Voice

Another Singer's Guide to a Short Career

Robert T. Sataloff, M.D., D.M.A, F.A.C.S.

Christina L. Mancheni, D.M.A.

Mary J. Hawkshaw, R.N., B.S.N.

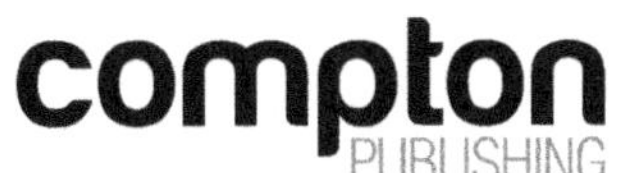

This edition published 2024 © 2024 by Compton Publishing

Editorial offices: 35 East Street, Braunton, EX33 2EA, UK

Web: www.comptonpublishing.co.uk

ISBN 978-1-909082-75-5

A catalogue record for this book is available from the British Library.

Cover design: Matt Oakley, Mojo Design

Set in Adobe Caslon Pro 11pt by Regent Typesetting

Contents

Preface

An article entitled "10 Good Ways to Abuse Your Voice: A Singers guide to a Short Career, Part 1" was written by the author (RTS) and published in 1985 in the *NATS Journal*, now called the *Journal of Singing*. The popularity of that article among singers led to the publication of Part 2 in 1986, and to the book *50 Ways to Abuse Your Voice: A Singer's Guide to a Short Career* which was published in 2014. Because so many singers found that book helpful, and because of many new developments in the following decade, a second edition of that book was published in 2024. It was written to provide straight-forward, accessible information to singers, highlighting common errors of commission and omission, and to provide guidance on medical issues that affect the quality and duration of an avocation or career in singing.

Recognizing that there are many more than 50 such "pearls" that could be helpful to singers, we are pleased to offer a new book entitled *50 More Ways to Abuse Your Voice: Another Singer's Guide to a Short Career*. As in the first book, we have kept the chapters and the book short and practical. The new book addresses many important topics and pitfalls that were not highlighted in the first book. These include the risks of failing to study voice pedagogy, anatomy and physiology; singing with jaw and tongue tension; failing to optimize physical condition and diet; pursuing the wrong career following completion of a voice degree; using body-building steroids; getting sick particularly with COVID;

not recognizing risks associated with some nutritional supplements; and many other topics.

We hope that our readers find this book practical, useful and enjoyable; and we hope that the knowledge imparted in these pages helps improve and extend our readers' careers as singers.

Robert T. Sataloff
Christina L. Mancheni
Mary J. Hawkshaw

1

Don't study voice pedagogy

Voice pedagogy, also called vocal pedagogy, is the art and science of teaching voice use including singing, and incorporates numerous topics related to singing and teaching of singing. It provides important information not only for teachers, but also for singers with no plans to teach (although it is common for such singers to change their mind and start teaching later in their careers). The study of voice pedagogy includes not only information on the art and science of teaching, but also knowledge fundamental to both teaching and performing. Components of voice pedagogy include anatomy (the structure of the voice system), physiology (how it works), respiration, support, acoustics, diction and articulation, registers, quality, vibrato, singing styles, voice classification, voice health and disorders, and other topics.

The importance of such knowledge to singing teachers is obvious; For singers who do not expect to teach, basic knowledge of pedagogy is important.

First, it provides the singer with information that is helpful in selecting a good teacher. There is sadly little quality control in the world of singing teaching. Although there are many superb teachers, there also are teachers who simply put up a sign or place an ad, hold themselves out as singing teachers despite having little or no background in the field, and collect cash for singing lessons. It is important for singers to know as soon as possible whether a new teacher is offering suggestions that are reasonable in light of what is known about the voice and approaches to healthy teaching.

Second, knowledge of voice pedagogy is extremely useful in helping singers analyze their own technique and troubleshoot voice problems (in conjunction with a good teacher). The knowledge acquired through studying voice pedagogy provides singers with a knowledge base and vocabulary to analyze their own voices incisively. Using such knowledge as a basis for singing and studying not only helps singers troubleshoot, but it also helps them avoid trouble in the first place.

2

Don't study anatomy and physiology of the voice

Any instrumentalist can name the parts of their instrument and describe their functions. If there is a sudden change in sound or quality, for example, a bassoonist will know immediately whether the problem is with the reed or something else. Unfortunately, many singers lack even a basic understanding of the anatomy (structure) and physiology (function) of the voice.

The anatomy of the voice is not limited to the area between the hyoid (tongue) bone and the suprasternal notch (top of the chest bone). Virtually all body systems are involved in voice production, but structures in the neck, oral and nasal cavities, pharynx, chest, and abdomen are central to voice production. A problem in any one of those areas can lead to dysfunction in all of them. For example, unrecognized asthma that impairs "support" leads to compensatory hyper-functional muscle use in the neck and larynx that can lead to vocal fold injury including nodules, compensatory tongue retraction that alters resonance and decreases audibility, and to other changes in technique that predispose the singer to voice injury. Similar problems arise if there are problems elsewhere in the body.

The vocal folds (formerly called vocal cords) form the oscillator of the voice system. They make a sound that is very similar to the sound of a trumpet mouthpiece without the trumpet. In order to oscillate, they require power from the "support" system which includes the lungs, chest, abdominal and back muscles, and other structures. Supraglottic (above the vocal folds) structures such as the pharynx, oral cavity and nasal cavity are responsible for resonance. The resonance system is largely responsible for an individuals' unique sound, and also for audibility over noise such as an orchestra. When problems arise in any one system, it is common for technique to change in all three systems. The task of a good laryngologist (voice doctor), speech-language pathologist, or singing teacher, or ideally a team including all three professionals and others, is to diagnose which system dysfunction occurred primarily (leading to secondary changes in the other systems) and how to fix it. The more a singer knows about how everything works, the better able they will be to describe symptoms and problems articulately, and to aid in rapid diagnosis and treatment, when problems arise. Such knowledge also helps singers recognize changes or imperfect function in any of these systems and correct them or seek care for them promptly before they become more troublesome.

3

Don't understand what your vocal folds are

While the vocal folds are only one part of the voice system, they are an important and delicate component. They also are more complex than they might seem to be to singers who have not studied the vocal folds from a scientific standpoint. The vocal folds are much more complicated than a layer of mucosa over muscle, as might be found on the inside of the oral cavity or mouth and throat. The vocal folds are layered structures including an epithelium on the surface; superficial, intermediate and deep layers of lamina propria; and thyroarytenoid (vocalis) muscle, among other structures. The epithelium and superficial layer of the lamina propria form the cover layer of the vocal folds. They move from inferior (low) to superior, and from posterior (back) to anterior, forming the mucosal wave. Even that motion is more complex than most people realize. The mucosa not only has to move freely and fluidly, but the bottom and top portions of the thin contact edge of the vocal fold move differently from each other, creating a vertical phase difference. Anything that interferes with such motion (such as swelling in the vocal folds, or scar) impairs the mucosal wave and interferes with the voice. The vocal folds and related structures also contain glands that are responsible for lubrication which allows the vocal folds to come together and separate easily. If the lubrication is not optimal, for example, if the voice is too "dry", the mechanical efficiency is impaired, and damage occurs to the cells on the surface of the vocal fold. There are two kinds of glands. Serous glands secrete thin lubricant. Mucinous glands secrete thick lubricant. They mix and balance to form lubricant of optimal viscosity. Many of the things that singers think are drying (such as some antihistamines) actually cause problems by shifting mucosal secretions from serous to mucinous predominance, increasing viscosity. That is analogous to having oil that is too thick in a car engine. It is helpful for singers to understand these facts so that they can make appropriate adjustments. Proper hydration helps maintain appropriate viscosity, and there are medications that can thin secretions when necessary. There also are numerous medications that thicken secretions and can cause problems for singers.

The vocal folds are extremely thin and delicate. They can be injured easily even by a sneeze or cough; but they commonly are damaged by forceful voice use with imperfect technique. If injuries such as vocal fold hemorrhage or mucosal tear occur, they may be followed by scar that leads to permanent voice dysfunction. Often, if such problems are diagnosed promptly and appropriate voice rest and treatment are instituted, complete healing occurs. However, if singers do not recognize the potential seriousness of vocal fold injury and continue to sing through it, irreversible damage can occur.

4

Don't get a baseline laryngeal strobovideolaryngoscopy

The vocal folds oscillate during speech at about 100 Hz (cycles per second) in adult males and about 200 Hz in females. During singing, movement may exceed 1000 Hz. The human eye is capable of detecting only 5 Hz. So, without equipment that allows slow-motion assessment, the condition of the all-important vibratory edge of the vocal fold remains unknown. Injuries to the vocal fold are common not only in people who know that they have a voice problem, but also in many others, especially singers (rock singers more than opera singers, but opera singers, too), actors, teachers, motivational speakers, football quarterbacks and other professional voice users, as well as many other people. Singers are athletes. Just as you would not be surprised to find knee injuries in a professional football lineman, it should not be surprising to find injuries in professional voice users. If such injuries are found only when a singer presents to a physician with a new voice complaint, the physician is likely to assume that the injury or other abnormal function is new and is the cause of the singer's complaint. However, often that is not the case. A great many singers (including elite operatic and Broadway singers) have abnormal laryngeal findings at baseline. These may include paresis (weakness), vocal fold cysts or other masses, reflux involving the larynx, hypervascularity (an increased number or concentration of blood vessels) and other pathology.

If such abnormalities are present and do not interfere with singing (that includes not causing the singer to use incorrect compensatory technique for the problems), then they do not require treatment. More importantly, they should not be confused with the cause of a new voice complaint in the future. Strobovideolaryngoscopy uses technology to examine the vocal folds in simulated slow motion. A baseline examination when the singer is healthy will identify such problems. The singer can be made aware of them and can record them on a cell phone so that a future laryngologist can see the singers' baseline examination and compare it with an examination when the singer presents with a new complaint. Having such information available to a physician examining the patient for an acute problem (on tour, for example) can prevent misdiagnosis, inappropriate treatment, and unnecessary cancellation of performances.

5

Lack good body awareness

Imagine the moment when you step onto the stage to sing – the spotlight awaits, the audience hushes, and your heart races with anticipation. In that very moment, do you consciously consider how you occupy the space (your presence), the position of your body; the tension in your legs, gluteus muscles and shoulders; your mood, or even your breathing pattern? Have you ever thought about how these seemingly small details can have a profound impact on your singing? Surprisingly, the simple act of having body awareness, or lack thereof, can affect substantially a singer's voice and how the audience perceives it. Body awareness involves attentively listening to your body, comprehending its functions and movements, knowing how it feels, and being mindful of your overall physical presence. Singing engages the whole body, and being more in tune with it can lead to better coordination of the muscles essential for optimal singing, and also can help singers learn to correct unnecessary (and sometimes automatic) habits and replace them with new, effective ones.

Singers who lack body awareness, or are yet to develop it, may struggle to identify and release tension in their bodies. For singers, comprehending and releasing tension, especially in areas like the neck, jaw, tongue, back, and core, is fundamental for achieving free, flexible voice production. Tension causes strain and fatigue, which can be taxing on the voice and cause damage if sustained over prolonged periods. Additionally, poor body awareness often leads to poor posture. Inefficient posture makes it extremely difficult to coordinate breath control and support optimally, which can negatively impact a singer's vibrato, resonance, articulation, and many other functions of the voice. Furthermore, a lack of proper support can lead to issues such as increased neck and larynx tension, "pushing" or "holding" the voice, all of which can have adverse effects on a singer's voice in the long term and can even lead to vocal fold injury.

Body awareness also can influence how a singer commands a room. Aspects such as a singer's body language (how singers carry themselves), appearance, attention, mood, body focus (back or toward the audience) and physical well-being all play crucial roles in singing and performance. A singer who is focused and presents with confident and expressive body language establishes credibility and command and can enhance the emotional impact of a song and make the performance more captivating. However, singing or performing while appearing to feel distressed, anxious, tentative, in pain, unhappy about appearance, or angry, can impact singing performance as well as singing practice negatively. These feelings and sensations can override a singer's focus and performance, and body cues that suggest such feelings can undermine performance even if the feelings are not really present. Singers should actively cultivate a keen awareness of their mood, focus, physical sensations, and pain level, as well as body cues that might project them to an audience, and shape audience reaction as this heightened awareness can help them identify and address voice-related issues.

Practicing body awareness can help singers become mindful of various aspects of their body, including their posture, breathing patterns, muscle tension, physical sensations, mood, and pain level. It also helps them to recognize and identify any areas of tension or discomfort and make conscious adjustments to improve their voice performance and overall well-being. Exercises, such as practicing in front of a mirror, massaging areas to release tension (e.g., neck and jaw), and reviewing video recordings of performances and/or practices, are invaluable tools for singers seeking to cultivate body awareness. Through these practices, singers gain insight into how their body influences their voice, as well as how they and their voice are perceived by others. By honing their body awareness, singers can unlock more efficient and optimal singing, enhance their overall performance, and prevent long-term voice misuse.

6

Sing with jaw and tongue tension

The human jaw and tongue are powerful. So, it should come as no surprise (especially for singers) that jaw and tongue tension have a profound effect on the voice. Although the main function of the jaw is to chew food, it also plays an important role in oral resonance and vowel sounds for singing. The tongue is also responsible for vowel shaping and sound resonance in addition to articulation of certain consonants (including /c/, /d/, /g/, /k/, /l/,/n/, /t/, /r/, /n/, /k/, /g/ and so on). The position of the jaw also effects the tongue and larynx (and vice versa); therefore, it is important to understand proper jaw alignment and tongue position.

Efficient alignment of the jaw occurs when the jaw is released and hangs freely from the temporal mandibular joint. This position also occurs at the start of a yawn. Simultaneously, the tongue lies gently forward with the tongue base relaxed and with the tip of the tongue resting effortlessly against the bottom teeth (incisors). Observing this movement highlights the important relationship the jaw shares with the tongue. Hence, tension from a jaw that is jutted, clenched, or tight adds pressure that is transmitted to the hyoid bone (which is attached to the tongue, floor of the mouth, and to the larynx) and base of the tongue, which constricts the airway, closing off some of the pharyngeal space and alters the shape of the resonance system. Consequently, singing with prolonged jaw and/or tongue tension commonly leads to several technical voice issues, and voice quality and endurance typically suffer. Tongue retraction, tongue base tension, and jaw tension also occur often as compensatory responses to medical problems such as vocal fold paresis. The extra tension is used to help force the vocal folds together, but it is counterproductive. It not only can lead to vocal fold injury, but it also decreases projection (audibility) by interfering with resonance. Jaw and tongue tension can be avoided through excellent medical care and voice teaching.

7

Don't optimize breath for singing

Breath is the foundation from which all great voice technique evolves. A singers' breath prepares the vocal foundation and will help, or hinder, voice technique and progress if not used efficiently. Singing is an athletic activity that requires endurance, strengthening and conditioning of the muscles (especially the core and respiratory muscles) and practice, similar to athletes. Although breath is an important part of singing, many singers (young and advanced) struggle in their understanding of how to utilize and take an optimal breath. Although the singers' breath is discussed at length by voice pedagogues in lectures, articles and books, many topics surrounding breathing for singing are still controversial and not agreed upon universally. It is bizarre that something we do naturally to sustain our everyday lives becomes difficult to explain when relating it to singing.

Because we breathe normally in our everyday lives, it is less complicated to begin (or think about) a singers' breath as an extension of (built upon) a "natural;" normal breathing. Healthy posture alignment is also critical for an optimal breath. Many of the muscles (diaphragm, abdominal, back and rib cage muscles) used to support posture also support respiratory function. It is important to avoid over-breathing, stacking the air, gasping during inhalation, pushing, forcing air in/out, and other methods that create extra tension in the body and restrict optimal inhalation and exhalation. Understanding the breath is a continual practice that requires dedication, study, thought and patience. An optimal breath for singing should be relaxed, flexible, free, and controlled when breathing in and breathing out.

8

Have bad posture, especially when singing or speaking

In previous chapters, we have discussed the complex interplay between the power source (support), oscillator (vocal folds) and resonator systems of the voice. The power source is particularly sensitive to alterations in posture. The effects of gross differences are obvious. For example, singing lying down is different from singing standing up. In addition, respiratory behavior (the way we breathe) changes when we lie down. However, more subtle changes in posture also affect the efficiency of support, as well as other muscle function throughout the voice system, including the function of muscles in the neck and larynx. Much has been written about optimal posture for singing, and it also applies to speaking and to other life activities. In general, the support system functions best with weight slightly forward over the balls of the feet, knees unlocked, shoulders relaxed, back comfortably straight but not "military," and with the chest and abdomen free to move without restriction. This should not come as a surprise to singers. It is an "athletic ready" position that is not much different from that used by a tennis player, a baseball shortstop, or other athletes. It optimizes breathing; chest, back and abdominal muscle function; and speed and freedom of motion. When optimal posture is not used, a singer has to work harder because of the consequent inefficiencies in the support system. As a result, compensatory muscle hyperfunction and tongue retraction occur commonly, and vocal fold injuries may ensue.

9

Don't prioritize sleep and rest

We live in a society that is constantly on the go. The continuous hustle to become a professional singer can be exhausting. It is easy to "burn the candle at both ends" while working to pay bills, auditioning, traveling, coaching, rehearsing, taking voice lessons, teaching, attending classes, taking care of family and doing many other things. These constant stressors contribute to our anxiety and increase cortisol levels in our bodies. Without proper rest and sleep, those cortisol levels don't go down as much as they should, contributing to a constant state of stress. This can lead to several health issues which will affect the voice adversely.

It is more beneficial to sleep and rest then it is to keep pushing yourself forward at the expense of your body's health. When we sleep and rest, our body and mind also have time to recover, de-stress, and heal. This is important not only for our bodies generally but also for the voice. It is difficult to sing while exhausted or under extreme stress. The muscles of the voice, as well as the muscles in the support system, are impacted negatively by inadequate rest. So, singers must learn to prioritize sleep and rest by ensuring that reserve enough time for sleeping and taking mental breaks. It is also important to do away with habits and routines that drain energy unnecessarily and that do not benefit the lifestyle of a performing artist. For example, eliminating mindless scrolling on social media, going home after a performance instead of going out to a late dinner, or taking a day off from work can all be beneficial in helping gain a few extra hours of sleep.

It is equally important to not over-commit yourself so that your schedule (work, personal or travel) becomes so demanding that you become mentally, physically and vocally exhausted.

A singer's instrument lives inside the body. Therefore, if the body feels tired, more often than not, the voice will be tired, as well. It is imperative that singers listen to their bodies when they signal for rest and sleep. Not listening to your body when it needs time to recover is counterproductive to the vocal and physical health of a performing artist. In addition, fatigue often is associated with impaired concentration, altered cognition, vocal tract tissue changes including dehydration, and an increased tendency to alter singing technique that can lead to vocal fold injury.

10

Use fad diets, and let your weight go up and down

For singers who struggle with weight (whether gaining or losing weight), it is not uncommon to try a variety of fad diets. The large number of fad diets (paleo, fasting, keto, Whole 30, vegan, Atkins, Weight Watchers, blood type diet, and many others) in existence makes it difficult for anyone to know what method works best. Each individual singer's needs are different from those of other singers. While a low-carb diet may work for one, a vegetarian diet may work for another, and so on. Diet or "lifestyle" nutrition does not have a "one-size-fits-all" solution. Therefore, each singer must figure out what works best for his/her level of activity and overall well-being. However, if the diet a singer chooses is not sustainable, it can lead to constant weight fluctuation which will adversely affect the body, mind and voice.

Living in a vicious cycle of gaining and losing weight affects the singer's respiratory function. It may also cause hormonal imbalances that can result in voice changes. If weight fluctuates too drastically or a singer loses weight too quickly, the body may experience difficulty adjusting to the sudden changes, and support and stamina will suffer. The respiratory muscles will not have enough time to adjust to the drastic weight changes, leading to altered support technique, decreased endurance, increased phonatory effort, and general voice fatigue. As more singers work (or are being pushed) to maintain and discover their optimal healthy body, it is clear that more adequate study needs to be done on the effects of rapid weight loss in singers.

It is imperative for singers to foster a healthy relationship with body and self. Because singers are athletes, what we put in our bodies and how well we take care of them directly affects how we sing. So, whatever way you choose to fuel your body, make sure it is sustainable, healthy, promotes freedom, flexibility and is enjoyable.

The authors understand that discussing weight for singers is a sensitive subject because it is hard to define the ideal body size or shape that a singer "should" or "should not" be. However, voice educators such as directors, teachers, conductors, coaches, and others often make comments about losing weight (especially for singers who they consider overweight). Efforts to make such comments are usually based on personal opinion or preference (not medical or scientific research) and often does more harm than good. The singer's overall health should be the primary focus as optimal vocal health goes hand-in-hand with optimal physical health. Furthermore, the topic of weight loss with a singer should be approached with the utmost care, as many singers have significant psychological trauma associated with this topic. The best encouragement for singers is to develop a healthy relationship with their bodies and to seek the guidance of a medical professional. Weight and optimal body conditioning are complex and should be managed by knowledgeable physicians, often in consultation with a nutritionist, exercise physiologist and other health care experts. This imperative for singers is no different from the needs of other professional athletes in the world of sports.

11

Don't work out correctly

Working out contributes to voice health as well as mental health, cardiovascular health and general well-being. The athleticism required for singing requires strong core muscles (abdominal, pelvic floor, gluteus and other muscles) as well as good aerobic condition and overall physical strength to perform in lengthy recitals, operas, musicals and concerts. Workouts vary and certainly are not "one-size-fits-all". Rather, every singer must find the most beneficial workout for his/her body.

Workout sessions should be designed similarly to singing practice (or lessons) in that they should be sustainable, tailored to your level, goal-driven (paced), have a warm-up and cool down, have a period of rest and recovery, and contribute to building healthy technique. Strenuous workouts that are performed with improper form (such as weightlifting, running, plyometrics, body resistance exercises like squats and lunges or performing advanced workouts as a beginner) can lead to body injuries that will impact voice health negatively.

In addition, workouts should contribute to breath (lung) strength and endurance. So, singers must be conscience of grunting or breath holding during workouts, as these gestures can lead to voice fatigue, hoarseness and/or vocal fold injury. Also, just as it can be easy for singers to over train (over sing), the same applies for working out. Working out too much (or doing too much before your body is able) adds unnecessary stress on the body which will affect the voice directly.

Although vigorous workouts have their place, singers often underestimate the benefits of a gentle workout for the body and mind, such as meditation, tai-chi, or yoga. A healthy mind is the foundation for a healthy body and for the voice. Singers require endurance, strengthening of the muscles, practice, determination, healthy diet, mindset and concentration, just as other athletes do. Since there is a direct relationship and balance that exists between the body and voice, choosing a workout that is comfortable, sustainable and growth-driven is important. Workouts should not hinder vocal progress or cause unnecessary pain and strain on the muscles that might negatively impact the body and voice health. Moreover, flexibility in workout schedules is needed to accommodate artistic demands. There is no reason to perform an exhausting 2-hour workout on the day of a major performance. However, good exercise habits are as important to the long-term health and success of a singer as they are to an Olympic runner.

12

Don't strengthen core muscles

Many singers often underestimate the profound significance of core muscle strength and its crucial role in achieving optimal singing. A strong core, composed of the abdominal, back, and pelvic floor muscles, is indispensable for maintaining optimal posture, balance, and overall physical fitness for singers. Moreover, core strength is a fundamental component of a singer's breath support system, which serves as the power source of the voice and the foundation for voice technique. As the core is connected to several essential muscle functions required for singing, insufficient core strength can lead to issues such as poor posture and breath support, resulting in voice fatigue, strain, compensatory tension, and potential voice damage.

Understanding the importance of core muscle strength and engaging actively in proper strengthening exercises can unlock a singer's voice potential across various singing styles and enhance voice endurance and control. This becomes particularly vital when navigating legato, staccato, and coloratura passages, and when controlling dynamics in singing. As core strength matures and increases over time, singers also are better able to develop the stamina needed to perform for longer durations of time, with greater ease and command over their voice, making hour-long recitals or 3-hour-long performances more manageable. Moreover, a strong core enhances overall body stability, providing singers with greater ease and control over their movements including hand and arm gestures, standing, sitting, lying down, and executing other stage directions.

A singer's training regimen should incorporate core muscle exercises that strengthen the abdominal, back, and pelvic floor muscles, being mindful to avoid strain or added stress on the body and particularly the voice. Forceful vocal fold closure, grunting sounds and other abusive phonation should be avoided while exercising. The singer's voice should not be hoarse after working out. By consciously engaging and strengthening the core muscles, singers can begin to develop a solid foundation to support their voice technique, maintain optimal posture, and achieve greater voice flexibility. Core strength should be combined with good aerobic conditioning and general health. Like any other kind of athlete, expert body condition is essential to a singer's success in achieving a healthy and durable artistic career.

13

Don't see yourself as an athlete

Many correlations exist between athletes and the singing artist. While many professional musicians are admired for their storytelling abilities, musicality and vocal technical capabilities that express a range of powerful emotions, the process from the practice room to the stage takes enormous effort. Singing not only requires physical and mental assertion as in sports, but it also requires muscle conditioning, dedication, endurance, proper nutrition, exercise, focus, development of skills and many other aspects that also are analogous to sports. Singers place many demands on their voice similarly to how athletes place demands on other parts of their bodies. Therefore, the muscles surrounding the voice, the respiratory system, and core muscles need proper conditioning, rest and training for a singer to sustain high level performance.

When singers underestimate the athleticism involved in performing, it can lead to under conditioning of the vocal mechanism and muscles required for optimal voice function and endurance. For example, have you ever tried singing after a long period of not singing? Suddenly, the phrases you once sang with ease cause you to gasp for more breath and the song feels like more work than it used to. That is because you're not in the same vocal muscular and respiratory shape that you once were. Athletes do not get up one day and suddenly walk into the best shape of their lives, ready for competition. Rather, it takes months and years of effective, tailored coaching and training. The same is true for singing artists. Lack of effective practice, conditioning, body exercise, nutrition, and discipline will undermine vocal growth. In addition, singers must work on their mental health and allow their bodies adequate rest and sleep. A singing career puts a great deal of stress on the singer's voice, body and mind. So, it is imperative to treat yourself and train like the vocal athlete that you are.

14

Take voice lessons from YouTubers

YouTube is one of a number of social media platforms that many people use to find out "how to" do or fix something. Because it is a free way to advertise services, many people create videos offering advice, even if they are not trained professionals or experts on a particular subject. In return, singers (or others) who are struggling financially (or do not wish to spend money for a service), may turn to these online "resources". There are thousands of videos online claiming to teach people how to sing (from kids to professional musicians).

Although it is great to have an extensive amount of information at our fingertips, a singer who seeks to learn how to sing from the likes of YouTube must use extreme caution. A YouTube video may provide incorrect or even dangerous advice or may provide helpful information on learning how to sing. However, those providing the video are unable to hear individual issues or discern if you are applying voice techniques correctly. This is a "red flag" since an important component of singing growth relies heavily on feedback from a voice teacher who helps you differentiate and understand a healthy, free sound versus an unhealthy one. Furthermore, inexperienced singers may be unable to sort through certain concepts that may not work or are too advanced technically. This is why most singers attend weekly lessons (particularly in the beginning of voice studies) at which they receive singing guidance that is centered upon their singing level. Learning too many concepts or advanced technical concepts too soon often leads to voice overuse and possibly damage. For these reasons (and others not discussed), it is imperative that singers receive voice lessons during which they learn at their own pace, gain a vocabulary and obtain expert feedback so that they learn to understand the difference between healthy and unhealthy singing, in order to avoid vocal fold trauma.

15

Take virtual voice lessons the wrong way

During and subsequent to the COVID-19 pandemic, voice educators and singers relied heavily upon virtual voice lessons to continue vocal progress. Virtual voice lessons proved to be beneficial in helping singers stay connected and encouraging continued vocal and artistic growth. They also have helped singers reach a wider community of voice educators and coaches (nationally and internationally) with more flexibility in scheduling. However, there are also some challenges associated with virtual voice lessons that may cause voice educators and singers to struggle with this lesson format, especially if it is not used correctly. For example, it may be difficult to correct/detect issues in posture, tongue and jaw tension, shoulder tension, knee position and other technical nuances that are easier to notice with in-person lessons. The audio feedback can be affected during virtual lessons, so a voice educator will not be able to play the piano simultaneously with the singer (something that is done commonly in in-person lessons). Additionally, the audio feedback may fail due to connectivity issues, which can lead to a cancelled lesson or incorrect assessment of sound. Furthermore, some pitches can interfere with the sound quality in many virtual platforms causing distortion of sound feedback. Moreover, singing and speech are sometimes altered when talking through an online device causing some singers to talk louder or softer in order to compensate. It may be difficult to recognize unsupported sound (especially if a singer is close to the microphone) or voice strain during virtual lessons. The size of the space and acoustics of the room also contribute to online sound and are hard for teachers to judge from afar. For instance, singing in a room that provides more of an echo (hall-like quality) may mask certain voice issues that could be observed easily in an in-person setting. Consequently, issues such as voice misuse, fatigue, and hoarseness could go undetected, leading to voice damage.

When taking virtual voice lessons and coaching, it is important to have the correct technical equipment (microphone, camera, internet connectivity, screen viewing) so that the sound quality and feedback closely resemble the quality of an in-person lesson. Optimal equipment is more expensive than the free sound and video used regularly for meetings and lectures; but the investment is worthwhile. Furthermore, voice educators should make sure to address posture and tension and be able to see the singers' full body on the screen. If that is not possible for the duration of the voice lesson, frequent checks should take place during the lesson to make sure that proper alignment is maintained. Virtual voice lessons can be helpful for the continuation of voice progress when live lessons are not possible, although they cannot replace easily certain aspects of in-person lessons; and both the student and the teacher should be conscious of the potential pitfalls of virtual singing lessons and should make every effort to avoid or compensate for them.

16

Rely on social media for your image

Performers are constantly being judged on their outward appearance. Even before singing a note of music, a singers' appearance plays a role in how they are perceived. Not only do we live in a culture in which what we see and hear (from celebrities, actors, magazines, books, movies, and others) enforces the idea that our image is what makes us "likable" or "valuable;" but we also experience it on social media platforms. The rise in social media platforms (such as Facebook, YouTube, TikTok, Instagram, Snapchat, X (formerly, Twitter) and others) over the last decade exacerbate this issue, and several studies highlight that social media platforms are causing a rise in depression, anxiety, cyberbullying, loneliness and other mental health-related issues. All too often users of social media are defining self-worth through the number of "likes" and "subscribes" they receive. The effect of social media comments (which can sometimes derail a person) can be profound. In response to the growing number of mental health concerns over social media, some platforms have altered the use of their like/dislike options, as well as the option to comment. Twenty-first century singers often are encouraged (by agents, peers, teachers and others) to post on social media to boost their audience reach. However, this can be a slippery slope, as some singers end up believing that they are as good as the number of "likes" and "subscribes" they receive. As the amount of exposure and reliance on social media grows, our sense of reality, mental health and self-value become altered. For singers, the processes of learning how to sing and developing and maintaining a career in performance already rely heavily on feedback and criticism, which are stress-inducing (not to mention the stress of performing in and of itself). Additional stressors from social media can have a profound effect on the voice, body and mental health, if a singer uses them for validation.

While social media has its benefits (helping people stay in touch, providing information about upcoming performances and ticket sales and other helpful things), the images and videos shared often are filtered, leaving no imperfections and also no resemblance to reality. Moreover, singing content often is filtered or at least biased on social media, as many of us only want to use videos that show us in the "perfect" light. This creates an unrealistic standard for singers to hold themselves to because everyone has vocal imperfections and days when they are not in "good" voice. There is a time and a place for a singers' best material to be released (in an audition or performance setting, or in a commercial recording, for example), but singers should not have to worry about being judged for the musical content they post on social media. If singers are constantly worrying about social media content, it leads to perfectionism, a trap that adds more mental burden, further adding to a false sense of value. Singers must recognize that the majority of singers do not walk around in performance dress, full face of stage makeup, with the perfect ensemble, and camera-ready in their everyday lives, let alone sing perfectly. However, even when we do have these things, they cannot drown out how singers truly feel about themselves. Therefore, it is important to embrace imperfections (acknowledge that they exist). Doing so will not only give you the opportunity to grow vocally, but also intellectually and personally.

No amount of "likes" and "subscribes" on social media will ever bring a singer peace if he/she relies on that to validate their image. More will be gained if the focus is shifted to an appreciation for the journey of learning how to sing and making music (being ok where you are), recognizing that there will be success and failures, moments of self-reflection and growth, frustration, break throughs, weeping, joy and a multitude of other feelings. Remember, your image, as well as your voice do not define you, but are merely a *part* of you. Judging yourself against the best images and performance that singers can manufacture for social media is unrealistic and counterproductive.

17

Compare your voice to others

Theodore Roosevelt once said, "comparison is the thief of joy." The numerous articles, books, TED talks, and research dedicated to the subject of comparison also share in this idea and reveal how pervasive the act of comparison is in our society. It is human nature to compare, but it can quickly develop into an unhealthy habit. Comparison is an addictive trap that can affect a singer's mental and vocal health, as well as self-esteem. It often leads to jealousy, envy, depression, anxiety, perfectionism, body image issues, burnout, and numerous other problems. It also removes the focus from the singer's individual voice, hindering personal vocal growth and progress. The longer a singer focuses on what others are doing, the less time the singer spends focusing on his/her own voice, and the easier it becomes to let comparison rob the singer of confidence, joy, and growth.

Many singers begin their musical journeys comparing voices, as many learn about music by hearing recordings or seeing other singers perform. However, the further a singer advances in a performing career, the higher the stakes become. The process of vying for gigs, competitions, university programs, young artist programs, and high-level opportunities leaves many singers fighting to get to the top of someone's list. Seeing colleagues garner opportunities you may want for yourself and comparing their success to yours can lead down a path of self-beratement and envy. It is fine for someone else's success to motivate us to work harder within reason, but it should never become the weapon we use to tear ourselves down.

Comparison among singers has become more prevalent in recent years with our culture's increasing reliance on social media, both for personal and professional use. It is not uncommon for singers (and others) to spend countless hours scrolling on social media looking through other people's photos and videos. What begins as an exciting way to connect and see what other people are experiencing can quickly become a time sink. While social media serves as a convenient and savvy marketing tool for many singers, the "peek" into others' lives also can become a trigger for negative feelings and emotions. It is also important for singers to remember that other singers typically put only their best performances and moments; and it is not reasonable to use those to judge one's own routine singing throughout a day or week. For most singers, it is best to limit social media exposure and, instead, spend time working toward their own unique goals.

It is easy to look at what other singers are doing and feel as if they are making more progress or getting better opportunities or training than you are. However, everyone's path, journey, and purpose for singing is different, and something that often looks desirable in someone else's life may not be beneficial for yours. Although it is difficult not to get sucked into the trap of comparison, avoiding that pitfall will ultimately give you more time to focus on your own vocal growth and opportunities. Singers should strive to focus on what they have control over, such as building healthy vocal technique and improving their skill sets (acting, languages, phrasing, endurance, and so on). This will lead to a healthy personal growth mindset. A singer cannot control what or where someone is doing or going on their journey, and spending too much time focusing on the things that are out of your control will only hinder growth, steal your time, sap your energy, and make you miserable.

Invest time in your instrument, embrace your journey, and learn to appreciate where you are. You can only control what you focus on and how you choose to navigate your time, so use it wisely and efficiently. Comparing yourself to other singers may not only add more stress to your life, but it will also negatively affect your mental health and well-being as both a singer and person. Every vocal instrument is a gift that is both unique and valuable (unlike any other voice in the world). It is the singer's job to discover what makes their voice special and to stay committed to discovering how to keep evolving into the best performing artist they can be. This does not mean that a singer should not listen to and learn from recordings and performances of great artists. However, there is a big difference between studying Pavarotti, Björling, Price and others for their artistry, and being upset with yourself for not sounding that good already.

If comparison is consuming you, seek professional guidance, and remove the contributing factors. Trust that you and your voice are important and understand that it is ok for your path to look different from another singer's. Being a singing artist requires vulnerability, and with vulnerability comes great risk. Practicing vocal technique is not enough. Singers also need to strengthen their sense of self-worth, learning to practice self-kindness and patience so that they can focus on personal growth and achievement.

18

Get desperate

The COVID-19 pandemic left professional singers (and other musicians) without work and a way to make income. This also stalled some singers' career progress, as some lost their break-through performance opportunity or important auditions (which were not offered again after the pandemic). As we move toward rebuilding performance prospects after the pandemic, some singers may feel that they must take every singing gig and audition offered. However, making decisions out of desperation instead of rational care analysis, can end up causing vocal harm or destroying a singing career.

Singers must recognize when a decision to take a singing job will jeopardize their health and professional growth. Sometimes it is more important to say "no" to an opportunity in order to preserve the longevity of the voice. Furthermore, as tempting as it may be to sing your dream role, attend a prestigious young artist program, or sing for an important agent or competition (and various other opportunities), doing so before a singer is vocally or mentally ready can add unnecessary stress on the voice. It can also damage a career. Critics have long memories for mediocre performance. Therefore, it is important for a singer to have a sufficient support system (experienced voice teacher, agent, and/or voice coach(s)) whom they trust to help them make decisions that will sustain, benefit and pace a career as a professional singer. If you do not have the correct support team that serves your best interests as a singer, it is important to find one that does. You should be able to trust your team to help you maintain perspective on your career especially when considering performance commitments.

19

Don't explore multiple paths after obtaining a voice performance degree

Many students graduate from educational institutions with a degree in voice performance and quickly realize that they are not fully prepared for a performance career, or that they may lack knowledge of how to navigate the performance business after graduation. While education in music performance (especially at the Masters and Doctoral degree level) equips students with skills in academic singing and writing, the highly competitive nature of music programs often results in many graduates leaving with limited stage experience, minimal teaching experience in a private voice studio setting, and they also may lack adequate technical proficiency and overall readiness for the industry. Consequently, after obtaining a degree many singers find themselves working in unrelated jobs such as retail, waiting tables, or other occupations to support themselves until they "make it." Some singers who have only a bachelor's degree choose to go back to school to pursue a master's or doctorate degree, only to encounter similar challenges after graduation. Thus, many students completing a degree in voice performance often feel unsure about their next steps after graduating. Such uncertainty can elevate stress levels and wreak havoc on a singer's mental wellness and hinder voice progress. In fact, many singers who struggle to find a job in the music field after graduating quit singing or begin to regret having chosen a path in voice performance altogether.

The journey to becoming a professional singer is often lengthy and demanding. Performing artists face rigorous schedules, exhausting travel, constant auditioning, rejections, uncertainty and the relentless work required to learn roles and improve technical proficiency. Additionally, some of the sacrifices a singer may make for a professional career can deter singers who initially idolized a performance career. Such sacrifices include limited time with family and loved ones, financial insecurity, extended periods of loneliness while on the road and many others. These realities can be overwhelming, leading singers to reconsider their dream of having a professional singing career. Fortunately, for those who have become professional singers or singing voice educators (or are training to become one), it is crucial to recognize that a degree in voice performance opens up a wide range of opportunities beyond traditional performance and teaching roles. This also applies to singers and educators who wish to work in the music field but may no longer desire to pursue performance or teaching as a career. Understanding the availability of multiple paths available within the music field post-degree (or during) can provide singers with valuable options.

A degree in voice performance opens doors to a multitude of exciting and fulfilling career paths beyond traditional stage performances and teaching voice. For example, such options include an artistic consultant, voice-over artist, arts administrator, speech-language pathologist and singing voice specialist all of which are excellent career options as are many other fields. By exploring alternative avenues after obtaining a degree (or during), singers can generate other streams of revenue, help evolve the landscape of the music industry, foster personal and artistic growth, broaden musical skills and perspective, and ultimately find the most fulfilling career for their lifestyle. Recognizing the diverse range of available options will empower singers to make informed choices about their future in the music industry. It will also help keep them from forcing themselves to pursue performance or teaching if they really do not want to. Trapping oneself in an unsatisfying career is not only unpleasant but also often unhealthy.

Additional career paths

Artistic Director/Manager	Opera Director
Arts Administrator*	Music Performance Counselor*
Cantor	Private Studio Voice Teacher
Church Choral Director*	Production Management
Composer/Arranger	Professor of Voice*
Conductor*	Singing Voice Specialist*
Event Coordinator	Songwriter
Music Critic	Special Event Singer
Cross-over Artist	Speech-language Pathologist*
Diction Coach	Talent Agent
Jingle Writer	Voice Coach
Music Therapist*	Voice Department Chair*
Owner of a private voice studio employing/supervising other teachers	

*Career options that may require supplementary education.

20

Don't be patient in building your technique

A beginner body builder does not come from the gym with bulging muscles after one session. It takes months or years of hard work, dedication, proper form, practice, balanced diet, patience, and many other disciplined factors for muscles to evolve. This process is also applicable when learning voice technique. Unfortunately, many young singers (this also can be true for advanced singers) in music institutions are encouraged to learn a wealth of repertoire for juries or recitals before understanding their own foundation for singing or having knowledge of some of the fundamentals needed for voice health and longevity (posture, breathing, free sound, relaxed jaw and tongue, efficient support). Moreover, singers are often placed into operas, musicals, or singing workshops to fill roles far beyond the singer's current capabilities. This enforces bad habits and can cause voice fatigue, overload and may be more difficult to correct over time. The demands of a voice degree program can add another layer of voice stress and mental frustration to studying singers. Unfortunately, sometimes academic institutions contribute to this problem. The best institutions assign roles to singers based on the singers' educational needs without regard to other factors. When that is not the case, singers should not hesitate to ask their singing teachers to help advocate for them.

Many institutions currently use vocal juries to test singers on their growth and progress by hearing how a singer applies technique through repertoire, languages, and musicality. However, reevaluation of this process may provide helpful benefits to singers who need more time to understand their technique. For example, a format that allows singers an extended portion of time to work solely on their technical foundation (including practicing scales, vowels with proper alignment, breath control and other aspects) before learning music will solidify technical concepts and behaviors essential for long-term vocal health and artistry. Additionally, testing of voice progress and function instead of repertoire requirements may help ensure that the singer is growing in their understanding and is able to apply methods correctly. Voice juries, as well as more demanding operatic/musical roles, can be given in the latter half of musical studies, so that singers can learn and perform them more correctly, safely, and efficiently. As voice educators, helping singers build a strong singing foundation first will affect the longevity of the voice and singing career. As singers, it is important to select performance material that can be sung well. It is better to sing "Twinkle, Twinkle Little Star" flawlessly than to prove to everyone listening that you have no business singing "Tosca," yet. It is also safer medically.

21

Don't practice properly

Practice is an important component of voice training, maintenance, health, and performance outcome. Regular practice helps singers learn about their vocal strengths and weaknesses, set and achieve goals, reinforce healthy voice technique, as well as develop discipline. It is often said that "practice makes perfect." However, if you are not practicing correctly and efficiently, that often leads to voice issues or reinforces incorrect habits. The understanding of healthy practice habits should start in the voice studio. However, some voice teachers encourage the use of healthy voice technique without discussing safe and effective ways for a student to practice technique or incorporate good technique into music.

Many singers go into the practice room and sing the most difficult passages in their music repeatedly, stopping only due to frustration or voice fatigue. This is why it is critical for voice teachers to discuss and ensure that singers understand what functional and beneficial practice is (this is especially true for beginning singers). It also may be valuable for a teacher to ask students to demonstrate how they warm up, sing and cool down in order to detect any concerning bad habits early.

Additionally, practice does not only pertain to the act of singing. For example, a student can benefit from mental preparation, visualization, obtaining a vocal track and listening to their part or playing their vocal line so that they can hear and understand (or memorize) pitches and music better. It is also important to work on character, rhythms, language and intent behind the music in the practice room. All of that can be done even when the singer is not feeling well or is vocally fatigued. Learning the music through silent study before attempting to sing it can save a lot of wear and tear on the voice.

When working on music or technique during practice, a singer can work exclusively on vowels or pitch onsets. Additionally, in lieu of singing constant high notes, a singer can sing down the octave until the song feels more secure (always with musical intention). A singers' practice should help enforce and build upon healthy voice technique, be intentional and time-efficient, and have several mental breaks planned. Because there are so many ways to map out a productive practice session, a singer should rarely leave feeling hoarse, vocally fatigued or mentally frustrated, as practice sessions such as these can lead to voice overuse, burnout and even vocal fold injury.

22

Don't manage your performance anxiety correctly

Performance anxiety affects voice production and performance by causing our bodies to go into "flight or fight mode." This mode, while necessary for alerting us to impending danger, can wreak havoc on our mental health and well-being before, during or even after a performance. It also can hinder vocal and performance growth. Common signs of performance anxiety include an increase in heart rate, dry mouth, sweaty palms, shaky legs and hands, nausea, upset stomach, memory loss, and many other symptoms. Although there is a variety of techniques singers can use to help ease/cope with such symptoms, management of performance anxiety is rarely a topic of discussion until later in a singers' musical studies, or after a singer already has quit singing. Unmanaged performance anxiety can have adverse effects on voice technique, performance and also a singer's self-esteem. Therefore, early detection of performance anxiety is crucial. Additionally, extra stress physically and mentally brought on by performance anxiety causes extra tension in the body, voice, support system, muscles surrounding the voice and other places. In order to avoid prolonged periods of performing in this manner (which will reinforce bad habits and bad mental mindset), it is important that voice educators and singers take notice of these symptoms as soon as possible and find strategies to help singers mitigate them.

Each performer must learn how to manage anxiety by implementing different methods unique to each singer's needs, as there is not a "one-size-fits-all" approach. For example, as our heart begins to race, we can take deep breaths to help calm the breath and body. Singers also can meditate, say confirming affirmations or use mindfulness before singing, helping to clear the mind of any unnecessary fears. Implementation of visualization techniques that encourage singers to visualize the performance outcome they desire are also helpful in controlling and suppressing fear. Additionally, as we see a rise in the promotion of mental health and well-being for singers, newer therapies such as Acceptance and Commitment Therapy (ACT) are being introduced to help singers with performance anxiety.

There is not a "quick fix" for performance anxiety and learning to manage with it is part of the art of being a singer. Most singers learn to function with performance anxiety and may even channel it to make performances more exciting; but some may suffer from debilitating performance anxiety which can derail not only performances, but also careers. For those who suffer from debilitating performance anxiety, it may be helpful to seek guidance from a licensed psychological professional to make sure that anxiety is not stemming from psychological or biological factors and to teach the singer techniques to control the anxiety. In some instances, a licensed professional may prescribe psychotropic medications to help with extreme cases of performance anxiety. However, such interventions are not usually needed and should be short-term, unless there is a problem other than performance anxiety that requires treatment. Singers must avoid abuse of beta blockers. In high enough doses, they suppress performance anxiety, but they also suppress cardiovascular response needed for the athletic act of performance, provoke asthma attacks, and lead to lack-luster performances.

More preventative education about performance anxiety is needed, as a career in performance already has high demands and stressors; and unmanaged performance anxiety should not be allowed to interfere with the quality or enjoyment of a career as a singer.

23

Take supplements without understanding risks

Singers are among the many people who use dietary supplements and herbs to maintain health or as alternatives to traditional medications. Because these substances are marketed as "food supplements and herbs," and because they do not require prescriptions, many singers make the mistake of assuming that they are safe. Especially if the supplements are being promoted through pop culture singing artists and mainstream media, that is not necessarily true. The ingredients in all supplements should be investigated carefully before singers ingest them; and singers should be aware that herbs and supplements are not all controlled federally for quality. So, they don't all contain what we think that they contain. Consulting a voice doctor before starting supplements is a prudent precaution. Also, when consulting a physician for any reason, herbs, supplements and other alternative/ complementary medicines should be included along with traditional medicines in the history that a singer provides to his/her physician.

Listing all potentially dangerous herbs and supplements is beyond the scope of this chapter. However, a few are discussed to highlight the potential hazards. Glucosamine is a very common supplement used particularly for joint health. However, it is extracted from shellfish and can produce a serious reaction in anyone with a shellfish allergy. Milk thistle, used for liver conditions, can have a laxative effect that can make it difficult or impossible to flex abdominal muscles in a way that permits effective support for singing. Kava, advocated for stress and anxiety, can produce not only gastrointestinal upset that also can undermine support, but also liver toxicity, headache and dizziness. Cowslip interferes with coagulation and can cause bleeding, just as aspirin can. Dong quai can have a similar effect and also alters hormone activity. Echinacea can be immunosuppressive if used for more than eight weeks continuously. Elder acts as a diuretic and can lead to dehydration. Feverfew can cause both dehydration and bleeding. Garlic, ginger, and ginkgo all also inhibit platelet activity and cause bleeding through a mechanism similar to that of aspirin. In addition to bleeding, ginkgo can cause G.I. upset, nausea, palpitations and restlessness. Licorice root, used as a demulcent to thin secretions, has estrogen/progesterone hormonal activity and also functions as a steroid and antidiuretic. Melatonin, which is used commonly to aid to sleep, also can have hormonal activity in some people and can cause immune dysregulation. High doses of vitamin E (4000 international units or more) also has it he coagulation activity and can lead to bleeding, as can willow bark. Yam, Yohimbe and other substances can have potent hormonal effects. St. John's Wort, advocated for depression, anxiety and seasonal affective disorder, can cause G.I. upset, photosensitivity, insomnia, anxiety and other side effects. Ephedra, also known as Ma Huang, is used to reduce weight and enhance physical performance. However, it has been associated with heart attack, stroke, hypertension, seizure and death; and this substance should not be used by singers. Ginseng is said to improve cognitive function. It also lowers fasting blood sugar levels and is used by some diabetics. However, ginseng can cause estrogen effects including vaginal bleeding, nervousness, agitation and insomnia. Horse Chestnut for varicose veins can lead to not only G.I. upset but also kidney toxicity.

The above warnings are not meant to imply that singers should not use herbs and supplements. Many products have been advocated for singers and not only are generally safe but also can be helpful. Actions of and reactions to many of those common products can be found in other literature,[1] and on the internet. However, information on the internet also is not necessarily expert or accurate; and singers should seek information about herbs and supplements from credible medical sites on the Internet, or personally from physicians.

The primary lesson of this chapter is that anything ingested, inhaled or introduced to the body in some other manner has the potential for adverse effect. Singers should not be lulled by the fact that herbs and supplements are readily available. Singers should remember that they also are unregulated, might or might not list all of their ingredients accurately, and have the potential to cause serious adverse reactions including death. So, singers should exercise diligence and caution before selecting and consuming herbs or supplements.

References

1. Sataloff, R.T., Hawkshaw, M.J., Anticaglia, J., White, M., Meenan, K., Romak, J.J. Medications and the Voice. In Sataloff, RT. *Professional Voice: The Science and Art of Clinical Care*, 4th edition. San Diego, CA: Plural Publishing, Inc.; 2017:1103–1131.

24

Don't realize that marijuana can affect your voice

Recreational use of marijuana has increased during recent years, along with the methods used to introduce it into the body. Much of the literature surrounding marijuana use discusses the effects of smoking marijuana with little mention on the effects of ingesting edibles or drinking it. With the rise in popularity of recreational use of marijuana associated with its legalization, it is clear that more education about the effects of marijuana consumption is needed in the professional singing community.

Most professional singers understand that marijuana alters cognitive function (some use it for this particular reason) but are often unaware of its effects on the voice. Smoking marijuana is the most common way to ingest it. However, marijuana smoke is impure and can be very harsh on the vocal folds and the lungs. Smoking marijuana not only interferes with fine motor control, but can also cause voice weakness, hoarseness, breathiness, laryngitis, and voice fatigue. It can affect pitch and overall vocal production. Side effects of smoking marijuana can result in irreversible vocal fold scar or other damage. While many singers understand the importance of avoiding marijuana smoke (smoking cigarettes and vaping), the effects of marijuana edibles and gummies on the voice are not as clear.

Some professionals believe that, for singers; edible consumption of marijuana is safer than smoke inhalation, but more research still needs to be done regarding edibles and other alternative methods of consumption. Research performed on the general population of edible marijuana users reports that general consumption of edibles comes with an increased risk of poisoning, as well as an alarming number of side effects.[1] This is due to the high and often unpredictable amount of tetrahydrocannabinol (THC) within edibles. Some of the side effects include sleepiness, respiratory depression, dizziness, hallucinations, paranoia, increased anxiety, panic attacks, agitation, heart issues, and dry mouth.[2] In addition to the vast number of side effects, edibles have a longer-lasting effect on the user than smoking. After looking at this list of possible side effects, it is easy to understand how edibles can negatively impact the professional voice user. For example, if a singer experiences dry mouth from edible consumption (commonly referred to as "cottonmouth"), the singer may end up working harder than necessary to achieve vocal fold closure and opening and also may have trouble maintaining adequately hydrated vocal fold lubrication. Although more research and education regarding the effects of ingesting marijuana on the professional voice user needs to be done, marijuana products in whatever form they are consumed should be used with extreme caution, if at all. Not understanding the risks and effects of consuming marijuana can lead to significant voice issues or permanently impair the voice.

References

1. Centers for Disease Control and Prevention. *Health Effects of Marijuana*, June 2, 2022, https://www.cdc.gov/marijuana/health-effects/index.html. (Accessed September 2023)

2. American Addiction Centers. *Marijuana Edibles: Risks, Side Effects & Dangers,* December 13, 2022, https://americanaddictioncenters.org/marijuana-rehab/risks-of-edibles. (Accessed September 2023)

25

Don't recognize that caffeine affects your voice

Caffeine, commonly found in coffee, tea, soft drinks, energy drinks, caffeine tablets, supplements, chocolate, and several other products, has become a staple in the daily routines of individuals, including singers. Caffeine is a stimulant that often is overused for its ability to boost energy levels and keep individuals awake. Caffeine also has a diuretic effect and can contribute to dehydration. Many singers do not pay attention to their caffeine consumption and are often unaware of the negative effects of overconsumption on both their general well-being and voice. Excessive caffeine consumption can lead to various side effects such as jitters, insomnia, headaches, upset stomach, increased mucus production, tremor (that may be audible during soft singing), aggravation of reflux symptoms, and others. Caffeine also can interfere with the body's ability to absorb calcium, which is essential for healthy bones, teeth, muscle function, nerve transmission, hormone secretion and other functions. These symptoms can make it difficult for a singer to maintain adequate voice hygiene, perform optimally or feel well.

It is important for singers to monitor and limit caffeine intake to help prevent adverse reactions. While the U.S. Food and Drug Administration (FDA) recommends a daily caffeine limit of no more than 400 milligrams per day for adults, singers with caffeine sensitivity should be aware of their individual tolerance levels.[1] An 8-ounce cup of coffee usually contains 95–200mg of caffeine, and a 12-ounce serving of Coca-Cola contains 34mg. Some singers may be more sensitive to its effects than others (especially those with medical conditions, taking certain medications, or who are pregnant). Caffeine also turns up in drinks one might not expect. For example, 12 ounces of Sunkist diet orange soda contains 41.5mg of caffeine (many people do not know that a healthy-looking drink like orange soda contains caffeine at all). That is more caffeine than is found in 12 ounces of Coca-Cola, but not quite as much as is found in 12 ounces of Diet Coke (46mg). So, it is wise for singers to check caffeine content even on substances in which caffeine might not be anticipated. Through incorporating caffeine-free options such as herbal teas, decaffeinated coffee, and beverages, increasing water consumption to stay properly hydrated (particularly important since caffeine can have a diuretic effect), paying attention to the caffeine content of beverages, food products, supplements and medications, singers can avoid unnecessary added caffeine and minimize unfavorable reactions. It is also important to realize that although decaffeinated coffee and teas are better options for singers with sensitivity, they usually still contain trace amounts of caffeine. For example, an 8-ounce cup of decaf coffee contains up to 7mg of caffeine.

Singers who are consuming high amounts of caffeine should reduce intake gradually over time to avoid withdrawal symptoms such as headaches, irritability and fatigue. Maintaining a balanced approach to health and voice performance involves finding the right amount of caffeine (which might be none) that supports overall well-being without sacrificing voice health. With awareness of the side effects of overconsumption and implementation of practical strategies to limit caffeine intake, singers can better maintain their well-being and preserve the health and longevity of their voices.

References

1. US Food and Drug Administration. "Spilling the beans: How much caffeine is too much." 2018. https://www.fda.gov/consumers/consumer-updates/spilling-beans-how-much-caffeine-too-much. (Accessed August 2023)

26

Don't clean humidifiers and steam inhalers

Steam inhalers and humidifiers are used commonly by singers to prevent dry mouth, nose and throat. Steam inhalers may help with edema and inflammation of the nasal passages, sinus, and of the vocal apparatus. It also helps bring moisture back into the throat which can help soothe a dry or sore throat, as well as provide relief from hoarseness. Humidifiers also bring moisture back into the larynx. While many singers use these devices daily, many do not understand the risks associated when humidification devices are not maintained hygienically.

When these devices are left unclean or not clean enough, bacteria, mildew and mold can grow inside them, become airborne in the humidified mist, and enter the lungs. This can lead to potential respiratory problems. Also, singers who use steam inhalers daily (or multiple times throughout the day) should consult their physician, as prolonged usage of steam inhalers sometimes can aggravate or worsen asthma symptoms.

Avoid adding essential oils when using steam inhalers and humidifiers as these products can cause or aggravate respiratory issues. It is prudent to clean and sanitize these devices after each use and perform a deep clean at least once a week for maintenance (to ensure optimal safety and usage, make sure to adhere to the cleaning directions that come with the device). Regular cleaning and maintenance will help prevent adverse health issues to the respiratory system and the voice.

27

Abuse corticosteroids

Corticosteroids are anti-inflammatory drugs and include cortisone, prednisone, methylprednisolone, dexamethasone and others. They often are referred to as "steroids"; but that can be confusing since they differ from anabolic steroids which are discussed in chapter 28. Corticosteroids are man-made, but they closely resemble a hormone that is produced in the adrenal glands called cortisol. Steroids can be given by mouth, intramuscular injection, intravenously, as an inhaler, and on or through the skin. They also can be given by injection into areas of inflammation such as knees, elbows, and the soft tissues of the larynx. Steroids suppress the immune system and thereby decrease inflammation by reducing production of chemicals that cause inflammation. This can help minimize tissue damage. Corticosteroids are prescribed for a great many medical conditions. However, regardless of the reason for which they are prescribed, side effects are common. Insomnia and gastrointestinal distress (sometimes including bleeding) even after; but other corticosteroid side effects include weight gain from increased appetite and other causes, mood changes, temporary psychosis, blurred vision, muscle weakness, excessive bruising, increased growth of body hair, facial swelling, acne, increased susceptibility to infections such as colds, worsening of diabetes and/or high blood pressure, osteoporosis (loss of bone); restlessness, water retention, eye problems including glaucoma and cataracts, and others. The likelihood of side effects increases with high doses and long duration of treatment. When steroids are given systemically for less than a week or two, most side effects do not occur except sometimes insomnia and G.I. irritation. Anti-reflux medicines should be used while steroids are being taken. Physicians try to minimize side effects by prescribing the lowest dose and treatment duration needed to accomplish the medical goal for each individual.

In singers, oral corticosteroids are prescribed sometimes for acute laryngeal inflammation. This should be done only if there is an imminent performance of sufficient importance to justify the prescription. Oral corticosteroids (or intramuscular or intravenous, which work faster than oral) usually decrease laryngeal swelling. However, there is no evidence to show that they alter injury potential. So, many physicians are reluctant to prescribe them unless a singer's technique and discipline are so good that he/she can be trusted to perform conservatively and to sing as he/she would have sung if the problem had not been treated. Inhaled steroids often are counterproductive. If steroids are needed for laryngeal inflammation, they should be given orally, intramuscularly or intravenously. Corticosteroid inhalers can cause laryngeal irritation and other problems. For that reason, they are avoided whenever possible even in patients with asthma; and in that population, only specific, small-particle corticosteroid inhalers are preferred. Nasal steroid inhalers used for allergy or congestion usually do not affect the larynx and can be used safely.

Unfortunately, some singers become psychologically dependent on corticosteroids and request them before every performance, or at least every important performance. Such abuse of corticosteroids is not medically justified and can be dangerous. Any corticosteroid use can cause at least some of the side effects noted above, and there is always some immunosuppression that can predispose to upper respiratory or other infections that a singer might be able to fight off otherwise. If a singer's vocal folds really are swollen constantly, then the singer should seek medical evaluation to determine and correct the cause, rather than using steroids excessively. Most commonly, such swelling is due to reflux, allergy or both; but there are other causes, as well. Corticosteroids should be used only under a physician's prescription; and physicians should prescribe corticosteroids for specific indications only.

28

Take anabolic (body building) steroids

Like corticosteroids, anabolic steroids often are called just "steroids". Anabolic steroids are man-made and function similarly to the male sex hormone testosterone. They include medications such as equipoise, winstrol, deca-durabolin, oxandrin, dianabol, anadrol and others. Anabolic steroids are taken most commonly by mouth. Legitimate medical uses include some kinds of anemia, low testosterone levels, loss of libido, endometriosis and other conditions. Anabolic steroids are abused most commonly by weightlifters and other athletes. Medications result in increased muscle bulk and strength. However, they are fraught with adverse side effects. These include hair loss and potential baldness in men and women, acne, growth of beards and other body hair on women, growth of breasts on men, decrease in breast size in women, liver tumors, occlusion of blood vessels in the heart that can lead to heart attack, violent behavior ("roid rage"), irritability, depression, shrunken testicles, reduced sperm count, lowering of voices especially in women (anabolic steroids are used instead of surgery in most cases for female-to-male transgender voice modification), bone tumors and other problems including death. When anabolic steroids are used by injection rather than by mouth or through the skin, the same risks associated with needle sharing in heroin addicts can occur in anabolic steroids users including hepatitis and HIV.

When masculinization of the voice occurs because of anabolic steroids, the change generally is permanent. The effect is similar to that experienced by boys at the time of puberty when voice change also is initiated by male hormones. Most of the time, people who use anabolic steroids do so knowingly. However, there are exceptions. In the United States, oral contraceptives (birth control pills) use either estrogen only or estrogen and progestin, not androgens. However, there used to be birth control pills with androgens, and they still are available in some countries. Singers need to be very careful about buying their birth control pills when traveling overseas and to make sure that they do not contain androgenic (male hormone) components. Endometriosis causes a variety of symptoms including extremely painful menstrual periods. Singers who have this problem need to ask about the content of medications that are prescribed either orally or by injection. They may contain male hormones. If they do, treatment alternatives (such as laser vaporization of endometriomas) should be considered. After menopause, libido decreases. While menopause usually occurs in women in their 50s, natural menopause can occur as early as the late 20s and early 30s. Treatment is available for women who want to continue to have an active sex life despite the menopause-induced decreased libido; but the most common medications for this condition contain male hormones. Alternatives should be discussed; and, if such medications are used, the voice should be monitored extremely closely. The long term effect is loss of high notes and improvement in low notes. Obviously, it is best for singers (especially women) to stay away from anabolic steroids or any other male hormone unless the use of such medication is medically necessary. For example, in older males with low testosterone levels, testosterone replacement with medical monitoring is reasonable and usually does not affect voice or health adversely. However, other appropriate indications are uncommon; and recreational use of anabolic steroids for bodybuilding can end a singing career.

29

Get COVID

The first known case of COVID-19 (coronavirus disease 19) occurred in Wuhan, China in December 2019. Worldwide spread resulted in a pandemic. COVID 19 symptoms vary from mild to fatal. They often include headache, fever, cough, fatigue, trouble breathing, loss of taste and/or smell, headaches, nasal congestion, runny nose, irritation, sore throat, diarrhea, shortness of breath, and severe acute respiratory syndrome (coronavirus two [SARS-CoV-2]). Symptoms become apparent from one day to two weeks after exposure, and at least one third of infected people have no symptoms. Most people with the virus have mild-to-moderate symptoms that might include mild pneumonia; but nearly 15% have severe symptoms. About 5% of patients with COVID-19 have critical symptoms including shock, respiratory failure and/or multi-organ failure. Older people and people with other health problems are at greater risk of serious disease and death. Some people continue to experience symptoms indefinitely. This condition is called long COVID, and it may last for months or be permanent. Long COVID symptoms can include respiratory (breathing) dysfunction that impairs support for singing, and partial paralysis of the nerves to the vocal folds. Damage to other nerves also can occur, including injury that causes hearing loss, facial paralysis and other neurological deficits that can impair or end a singing career. COVID-19 also can lead to seizure, stroke, complications of pregnancy including miscarriage, superinfection with fungus, and other serious problems.

The virus is spread by airborne particles. Appropriate masks that are worn correctly can be quite effective in preventing the spread of the disease. Although viruses mutate and new subtypes appear, vaccines and boosters have proven remarkably effective in preventing serious infection. Since COVID-19 infection can be a real disaster for singers, every effort should be taken to avoid it including vaccination and appropriate boosters, avoidance of people with symptoms that might be caused by COVID-19 (even though many people with those symptoms will have flu or some other condition which also can be problematic for singers), and use of masks whenever appropriate. The authors have seen too many tragic cases of singers with long-term respiratory impairment and vocal fold paresis (partial paralysis) that have ended their ability to sing professionally or even for fun. Virtually all of them have been in people who elected not to be vaccinated. There is no good treatment for many of the long COVID symptoms. Singers should understand that prevention is critical.

30

Don't give yourself time to recover from illness

When most singers think of illnesses, they think of upper respiratory illnesses affecting the larynx, oral cavity, nose and related structures. However, disorders anywhere in the body can affect voice production. Even a sprained ankle can alter posture, impair efficiency of support, induce compensatory muscle hyperfunction and lead to not only impaired voice quality and endurance, but also to vocal fold injury. Surgery of the abdomen, chest and back also cause problems with the support system due to pain that interferes with optimal technique. When singers undergo any surgical procedure that involves general anesthesia with intubation (placement of a breathing tube between the vocal folds), they always worry about vocal fold injury. It is unfortunately common for singers to sing a few scales even in the recovery room to make sure that the voice is functional, and to try to get back to performance as soon as possible. Performing with poor support can be more dangerous than not performing at all. After abdominal chest or back surgery, for example, a singer should be healed and pain-free enough to be able to do a few sit-ups (hopefully, the singer could do a few sit-ups before surgery!) before starting to sing again. The same is true following pregnancy and delivery.

Of course, similar precautions apply to recovery from laryngeal illnesses; but they are more known and obvious to most singers. They are discussed in more detail in chapter 31. However, like everywhere else in the body, the larynx and related structures should be given time to recover to baseline before they are subjected to the rigors of singing practice and performance.

31

Ignore voice changes with/after an illness

Voice changes that occur with an illness or that persist after an illness are not just inconveniences, they also are red flags. Voice change is a symptom. It is critical to know what is causing that symptom. Many singers tend to try to sing through/around a voice problem during or after an illness. That can lead to disaster, depending on the etiology (cause) of the voice problem. For example, if the illness was accompanied by a cough (or by continued singing during a case of "laryngitis") and a vocal fold hemorrhage (ruptured blood vessel) occurred, continued singing can lead to vocal fold scar and permanent hoarseness, rather than resolution of the hemorrhage and return to baseline. Risks are similar if the voice change was caused by a tear in the mucosa on the edge of the vocal fold. If the problem is vocal fold weakness caused by viral nerve injury, for example, singers almost invariably alter technique (often going from good to bad) trying to compensate for the problem that they hear in the voice and to maintain control of the voice. Such compensation is almost always the wrong strategy. Appropriate compensation and neuromuscular strengthening can be accomplished through treatment with the voice team once an accurate diagnosis has been made. Singers must remember to be smart enough to listen to what their bodies are trying to tell them. If a voice change occurs during an illness, even a cold, avoidance of heavy voice use should be considered at a bare minimum. If the abnormal voice persists for more than a day or two, consultation with a skilled laryngologist (ear nose and throat doctor specializing in voice) to determine the cause and appropriate treatment is advisable. That is certainly the case if the voice does not return to baseline when the infection has resolved. Medical care for singers has evolved to the point at which we can almost always help with such problems. However, if diagnosis and treatment are delayed, and especially if that delay results in scar that interferes with mobility of the vocal fold edge, restoring the voice to normal might be impossible. Understanding these issues and being gentle with a problematic voice until a diagnosis has been established and treatment has been recommended, can save a career.

32

Ignore symptoms of voice misuse

A common mistake among professional voice users is disregarding symptoms of voice misuse. The potential loss of income or fear of diagnosis of a voice issue can lead individuals to overlook or shrug off signs of voice misuse. However, ignoring these symptoms can have serious consequences that affect long-term vocal health and well-being.

Voice fatigue is a common indicator of voice misuse. However, many singers experience voice fatigue due to the demanding nature of a professional voice career, making it easy to mistake voice fatigue for general physical tiredness rather than the result of voice misuse. Other common symptoms of voice misuse include hoarseness (raspy voice), breathiness and pain. Persistent hoarseness during speaking should never be dismissed, as it might indicate an underlying vocal fold issue. Moreover, hoarseness can contribute to a breathy singing voice and require a singer to use more effort to produce sound. Breathiness can come from failure of the vocal folds to close completely. This may be due to many causes including masses such as nodules (which come from voice misuse) which hold the vocal folds apart.

Pain is perhaps the most significant indicator. It should not be ignored. If voice users experience any kind of pain while singing, they should contact an experienced laryngologist immediately. A voice issue such as pain is never something a singer should ignore or push through. Delaying medical attention for any of these symptoms could exacerbate minor vocal fold or other laryngeal issues and/or lead to permanent damage.

Ignoring symptoms of voice misuse can have serious consequences for professional voice users and can impact substantially the longevity of a singer's career. It is important for singers to prioritize vocal health by utilizing proper techniques, and seeking medical attention when symptoms occur in order to avoid the potentially serious effects of voice misuse.

33

Don't find a voice teacher who knows how to help you after a vocal fold injury

Often singers who present with vocal fold injury feel isolated and disregarded in the university and professional setting. For the singer who is learning to adapt to life with vocal fold pathology, finding a voice teacher who understands how to help is essential to the healing process and to building back confidence in singing. Unfortunately, many voice educators are limited in their ability and understanding of how to help a student who is recovering from a vocal fold injury. This is due to the lack of early education/training for voice educators on how to care for singers with injured voices.

A voice teacher who is unable to help a singer with a vocal fold issue could end up causing more harm than good including, but not limited to, a longer recovery period or more severe damage. A voice educator must have an ear that is able to detect subtle voice changes as well as a knowledge base of how to treat different voice injuries (not every voice injury will benefit from the same approach). Therefore, it is best for the singer to ask if the voice teacher has experience and training working with injured singers. Additionally, a voice educator should not hesitate to refer the singer to a more specialized colleague when the teacher's experience with injured singers is limited.

More training and workshops should be offered on vocal health and hygiene and caring for an injured voice during degree studies for singing musicians and voice educators. While there is a lot of useful information available through research, voice conferences, and masterclasses, basic training on care of an injured singing voice should begin early in the careers of both professional singers and music educators. Having or recovering from a voice injury is very stressful for the professional voice user. So, it is crucial to provide singers with the support and guidance necessary to recover. Singers should always contact their voice doctor and voice care team for guidance on selecting appropriate professionals before voice problems worsen.

Singers also should be aware that there are a small number of teachers who specialize in working with injured voices. They are called Singing Voice Specialists (SVS) and usually work with a voice physician. Many SVS also are certified speech-language pathologists, but not all. The SVS field was developed by the author (RTS) and Linda Carroll in 1981, and SVSs are now available in many medical voice centers around the world.

34

Use your voice excessively

Like any other complex neuromuscular system in the body, overuse can damage the voice. The anatomy of the vocal tract will not be reviewed in detail in this chapter, but the voice producing system involves skeletal muscles that build up lactic acid just as any other skeletal muscles do; delicate, complex layered vocal fold structures; vocal fold lubricant that has to be sufficient and of appropriate viscosity; complex interaction between the support, oscillator and resonance systems; and other features. Excessive voice use can result in damage through a variety of mechanisms.

When we phonate, our vocal folds make contact and then separate. Normal voice use often results in surface cell damage, and the body usually repairs that damage routinely. If the voice is used forcefully, loudly and for prolonged periods of time, and if vocal fold lubrication becomes dry or thick due to systemic dehydration or the dehydration associated with the frequent breathing that occurs during excessive voice use, damage repair can be impeded; and damage can become so severe that the body cannot repair it. Such damage may take the form of vocal fold masses such as nodules, hemorrhages, or other structural abnormalities. If excessive voice use results in hemorrhage, it may lead to vocal fold scar and permanent hoarseness. Scar also can occur following excessive voice use because of direct trauma to, or tears in the mucosal surfaces of the vocal folds. Such injuries are especially likely to occur if singing technique is not optimal and is associated with excessive tension in neck muscles and suboptimal support. When voice use is excessive, whether during singing or other voice activities, singers and speakers commonly fatigue and become distracted. When that happens, abdominal support often becomes less effective than it should be, and compensatory tension in neck muscles occurs commonly. This confluence of events is a typical precursor to vocal fold injury.

It is important to recognize that excessive voice use is not limited to singing. Singers sometimes do sing excessively (even classical singers), particularly if they are in competitive academic environments and participate in lessons, choirs, coaching sessions, performances and other activities. Excessive singing also can occur through agents who tried to book as many performances as possible, especially if these are paid through commissions on a singer's performances. Singers in high school commonly participate in every performance activity that they can find and use their voices excessively; and many of them have no formal training in how to use their voices in a safe, healthy fashion. Singers of all ages who perform pop, rock and other similar genres often use their voices excessively, particularly during rehearsals. They may rehearse in acoustically unfavorable spaces and sing loudly over music without benefit of monitor speakers or monitor earphones.

However, singing is not the only way to use the voice excessively. The same anatomy is used whether we sing or speak. Commonly, even well-trained singers use their voices to excess during activities such as waiting tables (over background noise), sales jobs, during athletic events as spectators or participants, at bars, at weddings or other celebrations, and socially while talking with friends at restaurants, in rooms, or on the street in open air with background noise. Excessive voice use during speaking that damages or fatigues the components of the vocal tract will affect singing; and attempts to compensate for those problems during singing may make them worse.

Singing and speaking are not our only uses of the vocal tract, including the vocal folds. For example, the vocal folds move and often make contact during playing of a wind instrument. When necessary, it is easy for a physician to determine whether the vocal folds are being used in this manner by passing a flexible laryngoscope through the nose and watching the larynx and pharynx during instrument play. Physicians do this routinely to observe the vocal tract of singers during singing; and the author (RTS) often performs such examinations on singers who play instruments to determine whether they have to stop playing the instrument when they are on voice rest. Instrument playing is often associated with excessive tension in the neck and larynx identical to that which singing teachers teach students to release. The better the wind instrumentalist, the less likely this phenomenon is to be problematic. However, many singers who play wind instruments for fun do not have extensive, expert training in wind instrument technique; and wind instrument use that is not expert can cause vocal fold injury. So, this activity should be considered another form of excessive voice use. These comments should not be misinterpreted as meaning that singers should not play wind instruments. Rather, singers who play wind instruments should receive expert training from a teacher who specializes in the specific instrument, rather than (for example) from a high school teacher who is required to teach wind instruments based on a semester course on the topic but who does not personally perform on or have expertise in the instrument.

Subvocalization is also a potential problem that can lead to hidden excessive voice use. Some people use their larynges and make vocal fold contact when they read. This also can be confirmed with a flexible laryngoscope that observes the vocal folds while the patient reads. However, there are other ways to get a reasonably good idea of whether this phenomenon is occurring. Most people who subvocalize are slow readers. They do not read silently much faster than they could read the same passages out loud. Furthermore, if they try to hum (which interferes with the vocal fold activities that usually occur with subvocalization), that slows down their reading speed and sometimes confuses them or makes it difficult for them to remember what they have read. Another hint is voice fatigue after a long session of silent reading. Speed readers virtually never subvocalize.

Like any other neuromuscular athletic system, the voice requires training to optimize use of the component parts of the voice instrument, training to increase endurance and a safe voice use time gradually, warm up and cool down exercises, and recovery time following voice use. Using the voice excessively for singing and non-singing activities can result in serious problems that not only impair performance but also shorten singing careers.

35

Sit wrong

Trained singers recognize the importance of posture, as discussed in chapter 8. However, most singers think about posture when they are standing to perform and give little thought to the topic when they are seated. People sing and speak a great deal from a sitting position. Long choral rehearsals are good examples; but singers also talk while sitting in classrooms, board meetings, social situations and in many other contexts. Posture while sitting is as important as posture while standing. However, while posture standing is pretty much under the singer's direct control, posture while sitting is influenced by the chair. There is a science to chair design and optimal seated position, and there are health problems associated with incorrect posture while seated.

The human body was not designed to sit with hips and knees bent at a 90° angle. Yet, many chairs are designed to produce that position, or an angle even less than 90° between the torso and the legs. The thigh bone (femur) can rotate only 60° in the hip socket. Getting to 90° requires 30° posterior rotation of the pelvis which causes flattening of the lumbar curve in the lower spine and creates torque on the back. This produces a C-shaped curve of the entire spine; and this position commonly leads to back pain through muscle tension, but also through increased pressure on the discs between the vertebrae, as well as stretching of the capsules of the spinal facet joints where the vertebrae connect. We can resist these forces and sit up straight using abdominal muscles, back extensor muscles and hip flexor muscles to overcome the forces that are trying to make the back slump. However, long-term contraction of muscles reduces blood flow to the muscles, causes accumulation of waste products including lactic acid; and these conditions typically lead to pain and muscle spasms. They also interfere with efficient use of abdominal and back muscles for support of the voice. In addition, flattening of the lumbar spine causes flattening of the diaphragm, limiting its efficiency for inspiration.

Use of a forward-sloping seat eliminates many of these problems. A forward slope of 15–20° usually is sufficient; it is unnecessary and usually uncomfortable to try to compensate for the full 30° pelvic rotation. The forward slope can be achieved by good chair design, or by use of a wedge pillow. In challenging circumstances, a rolled towel or sweatshirt placed at the back of the seat can help produce similarly improved posture. Kneeling chairs ensure good positioning with an angle open to about 130° between the torso and the legs, but they are expensive, difficult to transport, and may produce knee discomfort.

All of us spend much of our time seated, and we tend to relax while we are sitting down. Singers should be conscious of the mechanics and importance of posture when seated and should maintain the same diligence regarding posture and voice technique when seated that they do when standing. This advice applies to singers when they are speaking from a seated position as much as it does when they are singing. Failure to do so can lead to all voice problems associated with ineffective support, due to impaired mechanics caused by the posture imposed by most chairs.

36

Don't recognize the risks to the voice of airplane travel and of talking in cars

Airline travel is a regular occurrence in the career of a professional singer. However, it presents unique challenges to maintaining voice health. Several factors associated with airplane travel, including fluctuating cabin temperature and pressure, low humidity, background noise levels, and risk of germ exposure, can affect a singer's voice.

Airplanes are notorious for their dry environments. The air circulating inside the cabin initially comes from outside, and as the altitude rises and air is re-circulated, the moisture content decreases to about 5% humidity. This lack of humidity can lead to dehydration, resulting in issues such as nasal congestion, sinus pressure, dry eyes, skin, nose, and mouth, as well as reduced vocal fold lubrication. During a coast-to-coast flight in the US, the humidity rises to about 28% due to water loss from the people on the plane. For singers who may need to perform within a few hours or days after arrival, the effects of dehydration can be particularly bothersome. Singers should remain well hydrated and should consider wearing a mask which can help decrease water loss. Additionally, the constant background noise on an airplane may lead singers to speak loudly to compensate, which can further strain and fatigue the voice. The ambient noise level on commercial jets can be as high as 92dBA, loud enough to require the use of hearing protection in workers exposed to that level throughout a working day. To counteract these effects, singers should support their voices correctly and maintain good voice technique when speaking. Engaging in discreet voice exercises while onboard also may help alleviate voice tension and help maintain voice flexibility. Prioritizing sufficient sleep, relaxation and maintaining proper hydration before air travel is essential for singers. It is also important to allow time for voice rest and recovery, especially after long flights that may lead to jetlag, to give the body time to adjust.

Airplanes, as well as airports, are breeding grounds for germs, which can further impact voice health. In order to minimize exposure to germs, singers should continue to practice good hygiene habits before and during a flight. This includes frequent hand washing and carrying hand sanitizers to reduce the spread of germs. Wearing a mask also helps decrease the risk of infection, as we all learned during the COVID-19 pandemic.

The problems associated with speaking in cars are similar to those encountered when speaking in airplanes, except humidity usually is not an issue. Air-conditioning lowers humidity in a car, but rarely to a troublesome level compared with the humidity of outside air. However, noise is a factor. On a smooth road cruising at about 50 mph, most cars have a sound pressure level of about 70–74dB. There are exceptions, of course. The inside of a Porsche GT3 is just under 80dB, and the inside of a BMW 730d is a little under 60dB. There are other soft cars such as Rolls-Royce and Mercedes-Benz, and louder cars, particularly "muscle cars" and some sports cars. So, when we speak in a car, we are talking over background noise and have to deal with the Lombard effect (in which speakers increase their vocal effort when speaking in loud noise to enhance the audibility of their voice). However, cars introduce other problems. Car seats often have people bent at the waist to an angle of even less than 90° between the torso and the thighs, impairing support. If a passenger is talking to the driver, the passenger often turns his/her head at a sharp angle to look at the driver, interfering with the mechanics of phonation. This combination of factors commonly produces hoarseness and voice fatigue from extended conversations in automobiles. Long conversations on a telephone (hands-free or hand-held) pose similar problems, except for the turned neck position. Care should be exercised when speaking in cars. Seats should be adjusted so that the angle from torso to thighs is greater than 90°, and singers should use support, minimize loudness, and avoid extreme neck-turn to positions during conversations in automobiles. Some singers practice singing while driving, using recordings of scales or song accompaniments. This can be done without creating injury, but singers need to be extremely careful about technique, breathing, support and volume in the awkward environment of an automobile if they expect to be able to practice effectively and safely.

Understanding the impact on the voice of airplane travel on the voice and of talking in cars, and implementing practical strategies for voice care, can help singers minimize the associated risks, ensuring that they arrive at their destinations prepared to perform at their best. By taking precautions and prioritizing vocal health, singers can navigate air and car travel more effectively and protect their voices throughout the journey.

37

Don't cool down

Singers understand the benefits and necessity of vocal warm-ups. However, vocal cool-downs (or, warm-downs) are discussed and utilized less frequently. Since singing is an athletic activity that uses skeletal muscles, it is obviously important to warm up and cool down the voice, just as athletes do for their practices and performances (e.g., stretches before and *after* running). Muscles used in singing build up lactic acid just as other body muscles do. Vocal warm-ups prepare the vocal folds and surrounding muscles for the act of singing while vocal cool-downs help the voice return to baseline and prepare it for normal voice use.

Vocal cool-downs are beneficial for young singers, singers whose technique is not yet developed, but also are invaluable for advanced singers. Attention should be paid to cool-downs starting at the time of the first voice lessons. For example, beginning singers may perform technical concepts more incorrectly than correctly in the early stages of their career. So, after a voice lesson or performance, their larynx may sit slightly higher than normal. Therefore, performing descending scales and lip trills (or other exercises) for five minutes to cool-down the voice will help bring it back to baseline. More advanced singers find a vocal cool-down useful if they are learning a new role or are working on something that is particularly taxing on the voice, they may need adjustments similar to those of young singers discussed above. However, in any case, their muscles will have become fatigued and become lactic acidotic during use, and cool-down exercises are invaluable before the singer returns to speaking and other routine. The amount and nature of a vocal cool-down will vary from singer to singer. So, it is important to consult your voice educator(s) to figure out the best approach for your voice.

38

Sing in choir with poor technique

Many singers have a background in choir that began in the primary school setting long before learning about healthy vocal technique and hygiene. The choral art setting often requires that a choral music educator teach a diverse repertoire that covers a variety of genres and styles of music. In a single performance, singers may be asked to switch between different genres and access a palette of vocal qualities. Proper education of these performance practices also involves changes in voice production (for example, the use of "straight tone"). Choirs are exciting to listen to when they can demonstrate a range in dynamics and unified sounds. However, if the singer is unaware of how the voice works or how to support sounds in a choral setting, it can often lead to vocal overuse, fatigue, and/or damage. Both amateur and advanced singers will find that tongue or jaw tension, misaligned posture, poor seating, excessive volume, and poor breathing habits will detract from the choral experience. Proper education on various singing styles and vocal health is vital for any successful chorister.

Many classically trained singers are trained to produce vibrato in the sound from onset to the end of a phrase. Therefore, a skill such as "straight tone singing", in which vibrato is eliminated, can be taxing. In many education institutions (especially universities) in which the performers are training to become classical musicians, straight tone singing in choir generates frequent complaints. However, the use of straight tone for certain styles of music is common in a choral setting (although its historic justification remains controversial). Straight tone singing can be done without fatiguing the voice, but doing so requires efficient support and pharyngeal space. Squeezing the throat or forcing the sound will not produce adequate results. Another common complaint is blending. When choirs blend in a unified sound, it produces a pleasing effect. However, for singers who are working toward a solo artist career, blending can feel counterproductive and restrictive unless the singer has been trained in ensemble singing technique and unless the conductor understands the subtleties of placing singers next to other singers appropriately. It can also be difficult for amateur singers who are discovering their voice. Blending does not mean compromising technique. Rather, it is finding the unified vowel sound with other members in the choir to sound as one, and controlling volume and resonance as one would during solo singing. It is worth considering that most university voice majors spend a minimum of five hours per week "blending" in choir and only one hour or two in a voice lesson or coaching discovering their natural, free, sometimes rather *un-blended* sound.

In choral singing, all sounds should be supported and performed in a relaxed manner to not fatigue the voice apparatus. For example, soft singing (singing *ppp*, *pp*) if not supported properly can be misinterpreted as singing "off the voice," with extra air escaping through the vocal folds, leading to vocal fatigue. Sustained singing in higher ranges of the voice also can become fatiguing if not performed with optimal support. An expert choral conductor will be aware of unsupported sound and will help singers avoid unhealthy dynamic extremes in order to help prevent common vocal issues. Unfortunately, most choir conductors are not voice experts. Often, they are chosen as conductors because they play piano or organ. Instrument conducting technique can be unhealthy for singers; and only a minority of choir conductors are trained experts in working with voices. Singers should communicate any vocal issues or discomforts experienced in the choral setting with their choral conductor and, especially, their voice teacher to prevent singing with incorrect habits for a prolonged period. There is always a healthy way for a singer to participate in choirs.

39

Don't sing commercial or musical theater with proper technique (crossover styles)

Over the past few years, there has been an increase in the number of students wanting to study crossover styles, better known as Contemporary Crossover Music (CCM). "CCM" also is used to identify Contemporary Christian Music as well as Contemporary Commercial Music. CCM encompasses a variety of non-classical styles including pop, jazz, gospel, blues, country, rock, R&B, folk and musical theatre (although some consider musical theatre a category of its own). Additionally, there is increasing demand for singers to be more versatile and perform a wider range of genres and musical styles. However, many voice educators are not properly trained to teach CCM, as most educational institutions still only offer programs that utilize either the Western Classical tradition or musical theatre techniques. Even in institutions that offer both Western Classical and musical theatre programs, students often are not given easy access to train in both programs. The lack of educational institutions offering voice training in CCM technique and voice health often requires singers to either seek training outside of the university setting or to try to figure it out on their own. Therefore, it is imperative to find a voice educator who not only has expertise in classical technique, but also in singing and teaching CCM technique (or is willing to refer you to a trusted colleague who teaches CCM technique, if it is beyond your primary teacher's expertise).

CCM technique requires a different vocal approach to sound, and each style requires a different set of vocal skills and production. For example, CCM styles often utilize more chest voice, belting, speech-like sound, straight-tone, and a variety of other voice textures and colors. Additionally, some CCM styles may change the shape of the vocal tract and position of the larynx (slightly raised) to achieve different voice qualities. Whereas classical technique requires balanced registers of the head and chest, a relaxed, low larynx, an elongated vocal tract, a consistently raised soft palate and tall vowels, and vibrato in every note, contemporary styles do not rely on these techniques, and often employ technical choices that are the opposite of what a classically trained singer would choose. It is possible to achieve these CCM aesthetics in a safe and healthy fashion, especially since CCM singers usually use an amplifier rather than trying to project their voice to fill a 2000-seat theater. If the voice educator or singer lacks the necessary training in CCM styles, that can lead to vocal overuse, burnout, and voice damage – not to mention a sound that is inconsistent with the style of the song in question.

CCM styles can be complicated or difficult to master (especially if you are re-training from a classical approach), and nuanced technical concepts inherent to the style are often misunderstood when approached from a classical perspective (such as belting, which is often misinterpreted as "pushing" or "yelling"). Also, singing loudly in order to sound more "powerful" can lead to forcing the larynx too high, straining, or yelling--all of which are hard on the vocal folds. Additionally, as noted above, CCM is always performed with a mic, something that many classical singers don't even consider, as they are taught to amplify their sound through resonance and shaping of the vocal tract. Use of a microphone and amplifier requires training and is not as simple as just singing into an amplification system. CCM styles can be performed in a healthy way as long as the voice educator and singer understand how to develop the voice to perform the singing functions necessary in a way that it is flexible, supported, and free. Voice educators and singers working on CCM technique must be able to discern the dangers of improper contemporary technique. More programs offering courses in CCM pedagogy also may help bridge the gap between styles so that singers leave educational institutions as multifaceted artists. Proper education of vocal cross-training with functional technique will help singers avoid some of the common pitfalls of this style that lead to voice fatigue and injury.

40

Don't mark correctly

Marking is a singing technique used to preserve (not add vocal stress to) the voice during a typically long period of singing (used particularly during staging rehearsals or in voice coaching), during which a performer will sing with "half voice" (using less vocal intensity, eliminating very high and low notes, and not singing or speaking except when necessary). It can be taxing on the voice to sing out during hours' worth of rehearsals or voice coaching. Additionally, singers may choose to mark when they are not in "good" voice.

Although marking is a common technical practice, many singers do not know how to mark appropriately, leading to voice overuse or damage rather than rest and protection. So, it is important to learn how to mark under the tutelage of a voice teacher and to incorporate marking into your practice. Marking does not mean sing "off" the voice. Rather, marking requires a healthy, supported voice production and character intention. While marking, a singer can alter pitches and singing volume (dynamics). For example, higher pitches can be performed an octave lower (or in falsetto for male voices). Performers should be technically secure in whatever they sing before incorporating marking. This will make it easier for singers to map out where they plan to mark their music, thus avoiding vocal surprises for themselves. While marking is beneficial, doing so incorrectly can impact vocal health negatively.

41

Choose an institution for its prestige instead of for the voice teacher

Juilliard, Curtis, Academy of Vocal Arts, Peabody (and many others), are well known to singers as the most coveted and prestigious institutions for aspiring professional singers. However, going to a reputable or prestigious institution does not guarantee that you will graduate as the best singer that you could be, or with a sophisticated understanding of how your voice functions or with several performances on your resume. While prestigious singing institutions may offer allure and recognition, the expertise and guidance of a skilled voice teacher are fundamental to a singer's technical, artistic, and professional development. In addition, finding a high-quality voice teacher who can provide tailored instruction to address the specific needs and goals of a singer can help the singer avoid voice misuse and make the training process less stressful. While prestigious institutions often have excellent voice teachers, they also sometimes have a famous singer on the faculty who may be a better singer than teacher. Singers should shift their focus to finding a voice teacher whose pedagogical expertise, career knowledge base, teaching style, and care can effectively guide them toward a successful career. If they happen to be at a famous institution, so much the better; but the quality of teaching received during years of training is more important for singers seeking a performance career than the name of the school.

In addition, having an excellent voice teacher is far more beneficial to a singer than enduring the stress and potential negative impact on voice health and overall well-being that can arise from dealing with an unhelpful voice teacher at a prestigious institution and trying to switch to a new voice teacher within that institution (or going through the process of finding a new teacher and/or school).

It is important to seek recommendations for voice teachers at different institutions and to interview and have a lesson with potential voice teachers so that you can access teaching style and compatibility. The voice teacher a singer chooses should not only have qualities that align with the singer's personal and professional goals but also understand how to nurture talent. Singers should access the institution's culture by learning about possible performance opportunities, curriculum, facilities, faculty and staff, support, student rapport, financial resources, and the activities and success history of previous graduates/trainees. However, the voice teacher should be the primary focus of an institution search. By prioritizing the quality of voice instruction over prestige alone, singers can lay a solid foundation for their vocal development and increase their chances of achieving long-term success in their careers. Optimal training also will minimize the risks of vocal fold injury and other preventable health problems.

42

Don't recognize lung problems

Most singers are familiar with the term "support". It refers to function of the power source of the voice that generates a controlled air stream that passes between the vocal folds and allows phonation. Singing teachers help their students develop strength and control the muscles of the chest, abdomen, back and related structures so that singers can create a consistent flow of air below and between the vocal folds. When the power source is not functioning optimally, singers typically compensate by recruiting delicate muscles in the neck that are not designed for power functions. That common but inefficient strategy leads not only to problems in the quality and control of the singing voice, but also sometimes to vocal fold injury and even masses that may require surgery. The most common cause of inadequate support is improper technique. However, that is not the only cause. Respiratory (breathing) abnormalities can undermine support even when a singer's technique is flawless. They also cause similar problems in and consequences for wind instrumentalists. For singers who also play wind instruments, vocal fold injury acquired during one activity will create problems that cross over into the other musical activity.

While severe breathing problems such as those that can occur with a bad respiratory infection such as pneumonia are obvious, even mild respiratory problems can have major consequences for the voice. For this reason, we have performed lung screening on nearly every new voice patient for decades. It is astounding how often we find treatable abnormalities of which the patient was unaware. For example, even mild asthma can have major impact. Asthma involves bronchospasm. That is, it causes the airways to close down. So, even if all the muscles of support are working effectively, airflow is capped by the airway spasm, and an optimal air stream cannot be delivered to the vocal folds. Such patients have technical difficulties including tongue retraction (throaty singing, or pressed phonation). That problem is common among singers, but in patients with asthma and other lung problems, there is a medical reason for it. Once the asthma is treated, technique often improves immediately. To make matters worse, asthma can often be induced by exercise; and singing is a form of exercise. Exercise-induced asthma even in runners is caused by drying of the airway. During a concert, singers not only exercise, sweat and dehydrate, but they also breathe frequently, sometimes under hot lights. So, it should not be surprising that exercise-induced asthma can be caused by the exercise of singing.

There are many other lung problems that also can undermine support. They include even mild chronic obstructive lung disease that is most common in smokers, and restrictive lung disease that is seen most often in obese people. There are also many other common medical conditions that can affect the lungs adversely, including reflux from the stomach with chronic aspiration into the lungs. That can even lead to lung damage that can be seen on x-ray studies and that decreases the effectiveness of the lungs, sometimes permanently.

If singers seem to have less "breath" than they think that they should when exercising, even when walking upstairs, lung problems should be suspected, although such problems can be due just to being out of shape. Being "out of shape" usually means poor aerobic conditioning. Singers are vocal athletes, and they depend upon good aerobic conditioning and core muscle strength for the support necessary for healthy phonation. However, even when there is no obvious shortness of breath, singers who have difficulty releasing tongue base tension and other muscle hyperfunction should consider the possibility that they are not just challenged learners in the studio but rather are compensating for an unrecognized medical problem. Suboptimal lung function is a common one, although there are many others such as vocal fold weakness (paresis). We test for lung problems even when there are no obvious symptoms. Certainly, if singers suspect that there may be a medical reason for support difficulties, obtaining pulmonary function tests is easy and painless. It is important that they be interpreted correctly, however. If pulmonary function tests are at the low end of normal or mildly abnormal in a trained singer, most doctors will assume that they are fine; but they are not. Doctors would recognize a problem if the singer were an Olympic runner, but unfortunately most doctors are not as attuned to the fact that various aspects of lung function should be better than normal in singers, just as they should in other athletes. Failure to recognize and treat even minor lung dysfunction can limit a singing career severely.

43

Ignore pollution

Environmental pollution occurs everywhere. In some cities, it is worse than others; but we encounter it inside and outside almost everywhere. Many pollutants damage the voice. Some do so directly by causing irritation of the mucosa of the vocal folds and resonator system. Pollutants can interfere with lung function, undermining support. Singers should be aware of problems associated with pollution and try to avoid exposures whenever possible, or at least minimize them.

Atmospheric pollution is the best recognized form. Consequences are obvious in severe cases such as when people are exposed to industrial accidents, fires or other adverse events that cause severe inflammation of the respiratory passages from the nose through the lungs. Usually, the consequences of such insults are temporary; but sometimes they are permanent. Similar problems can occur slowly from more subtle exposures to environmental pollutants which exist in practically every city. In some cases, the mechanisms are obvious, especially when someone has coughed from the pollution and sustained a vocal fold hemorrhage or tear, when there has been a burn, or when mucosal inflammation is severe. When pollution is troublesome enough to cause cough, it often also decreases lung function and impairs support, leading to other problems from attempts at compensation.

Performing artists encounter special problems with pollution. These include exposure to dust from curtains that have not been clean for years, inhalation of sawdust and aspiration of fumes from construction of flats during rehearsals (not an issue for elite performers, but common in amateur and community theater), and exposure to stage fog, stage smoke and pyrotechnics. Lipoid-based fogs create wonderful effects because the suspended oil droplets diffract light beautifully. Unfortunately, when singers and actors inhale the oil droplets, they can stay in the lungs permanently and cause serious lung dysfunction over time. Glycol-based fogs cause mucosal irritation, but they usually do not result in permanent damage unless the irritation is severe enough to cause cough and vocal fold injury. Pyrotechnics used to be used only outdoors, but that is no longer the case. Frequent exposure to pyrotechnics is associated not only with the topical irritation common to other stage effects, but also with serious neurological injury. The colors in pyrotechnic effects are created by vaporizing heavy metals. For example, the green color comes from copper. Heavy metals are neurotoxic; that is, they damage nerves. There also are other substances that can be inhaled in theaters and other older buildings that can cause serious, permanent injury. Asbestos is a classic example, but even mold can be problematic. Singers need to be very careful about controlling such exposures.

Although we will not discuss them in detail, there are also pollutants that are not inhaled. They can be ingested or acquired through skin absorption, for example. Some of these also can provoke respiratory reactions, and some of them are neurotoxic.

It is prudent for singers to be familiar with the hazards associated with exposures to certain pollutants and to avoid them whenever possible, even if that means passing up a job because it is associated with high risk that cannot be eliminated through alternatives or controlled through negotiation with management.

44

Sing in masks

A great deal of more research is needed to learn everything that we need to know about singing with masks. However, nearly all singers have had to sing with masks during the pandemic, and it is likely that we will need to sing with masks intermittently in the future. On the one hand, masks are quite effective at protecting singers from serious illnesses such as COVID-19 which can end a singing career, as discussed in chapter 29, and they also provide protection against flu and the common cold. Physicians saw far fewer patients with colds during the pandemic than we did before or after. On the other hand, masks create resistance to breathing which can cause fatigue. Moreover, the better the mask is at protecting against aerosol exposure, the more resistance to breathing it creates even if the mask is held off the nose and mouth by design or by a plastic spacer. For example, it is much easier to breathe through a cloth mask than through an N-95 respirator, but the N-95 provides superior protection against infection. Masks also often restrict jaw motion leading singers to compensate with extra effort. Extra effort also can occur because of acoustic effects. Low notes are softer when sung through a mask, and there can be effects on higher notes, as well, depending on the material that was used to make the mask. Singers who recognize this may try to compensate, and choral conductors may call for more sound to compensate, which can leave singers fatigued by the end of a rehearsal. If a singer is hoarse or fatigued, or if the range and dynamic control of the voice have diminished after singing, then something happened during singing that should not have happened. In some cases, the voice changes are due to efforts to compensate for the effects of the mask. When singers must wear masks, they should sing exactly as they would have sung if they were not wearing them.

A problem that has not been discussed adequately is the effect of hiding the mouth and tongue behind a mask. When conductors, teachers, colleagues and other critics cannot see a singer's mouth and tongue, jaw tension and tongue tension may go unnoticed and uncorrected, especially when the singer is working against the mask physically during mouth opening. Most singing lessons, even during the pandemic, have been conducted without masks virtually, and often without masks in person. If singers are going to have to sing with masks, their teachers should spend some lesson time with them singing with masks on to be certain that technique remains good despite the mask, and to identify consequences of the mask in each individual singer that are likely to lead to adverse changes in singing technique.

45

Don't recognize that your gender can affect vocal fold pathology and treatment

It would be nice to think that gender is irrelevant to voice disorders and treatment; but that is not the case. Males and females develop somewhat different voice pathology problems.

For example, specifically with reference to masses on the vocal folds, nodules are more common in women (and children) than they are in adult men. A mass (such as a cyst) on one vocal fold often causes a reactive mass from contact trauma on the other vocal fold. Reactive masses are more common in women than in men. Females also are more likely than males to have a pseudocyst, a fluid-filled lesion without a capsule (true cysts have capsules). The consequences of masses also differ by gender. Females are more likely to have high shimmer values (perturbations, or variations, in intensity) and abnormally low maximum phonation times (ability to hold a note) compared with men. Most experts agree that the best treatment for vocal fold masses is voice therapy, followed by surgery if therapy is not sufficient for the singer. Interestingly, women are more likely to be willing to participate in therapy than men, although the difference in adherence to therapy is less among professional singers than it is in the general population.

While vocal fold masses are among the more serious problems that can affect singers, there are many more common voice problems, and they also are associated with gender differences. For example, teachers are among the professional voice users with the highest voice demands. Compared to vocally healthy adults in other professions, teachers are three times more likely to experience voice fatigue, physical discomfort from voice use, and to avoid voice use when possible. Female teachers are substantially more likely than males to have Vocal Fatigue Index (VFI) scores approaching the level considered abnormal (the presence of dysphonia) than men. Similar patterns occur in call-center personnel and other professional voice users.

Although more study is needed, it appears that these medical issues are compounded by societal perception. Most people are less likely to notice or be bothered by voice abnormalities in men than in women. The intolerance of dysphonia in women (often unconscious bias) may have more adverse effects than generally recognized in many areas, including job placement.

Although in the current era of political correctness it would be comforting to believe that there is no difference between men and women with reference to voice pathology, medical care, and real-life consequences of voice abnormalities, that does not appear to be the case. Singers should be aware of medical differences and unconscious biases; and all of us should encourage further study of this complex issue to improve diagnosis, treatment and public education.

46

Don't recognize endocrine (hormone) disorders' voice risks

The voice is extremely sensitive to even minor fluctuations in the body's hormone environment. Some endocrine (hormone) voice effects are physiologic (normal). The most prominent and well-known involves sex hormones. They are responsible for voice change at the time of puberty, for example, and that is a physiologic process. When voice change fails to occur especially in males, the voice can remain soprano, a condition known as puberphonia. That can occur either with other failures of maturation, or in the presence of normal secondary sex characteristics in all other body systems. Generally, voice change in males and females should begin starting at age 12 to 17. If puberty has not started by then, it is considered delayed. During puberty, male voices drop about one octave, and female voices usually drop about one third of an octave. Failure of the voice to change, or changes that are substantially outside expected parameters, warrant medical evaluation.

The menstrual cycle also involves physiologic hormone-induced voice changes. About one third of women experience premenstrual decrease in voice efficiency, loss of high notes, slight hoarseness, voice fatigue, slight muffling of the voice and other symptoms. Nearly as many experience the same symptoms for a day or two immediately before ovulation. Especially before menses, the voice changes may be associated with blood vessel changes that increase the risk of hemorrhage. That risk is even greater if support is impaired by painful menstrual cramps, and especially if medicine that promotes bleeding (such as aspirin and ibuprofen, as well as others discussed in chapter 47) has been taken to ease the discomfort caused by cramps. While cyclical voice changes are routine for some women, if they are incapacitating, physicians often can provide help. Pregnancy also causes voice changes both through hormone-induced alterations in the vocal folds, and through mechanical impairment of support, especially late in pregnancy.

About 25% of women reach menopause before age 45, and 95% do so by the age of 55. After menopause, the ovaries secrete less estrogen but continue to produce androgens (male hormones). Without estrogen to oppose the androgen effect, female voices drop gradually over the decades following menopause. Such changes can be prevented or minimized by hormone replacement which should be considered when there is no medical contraindication. They also are less prominent in trained professional singers than in people with untrained voices.

Sex hormone problems also used to be quite common with birth control pills. However, modern, low-estrogen birth control pills that contain no androgens generally do not cause adverse voice changes. In fact, some research has shown that they result in voice improvement. Nevertheless, women starting oral contraception should monitor their voices carefully so that the medications can be stopped or changed if voice alterations occur. Most such changes are reversible. However, the voice changes caused by androgens (male hormones) used for endometriosis, diminished libido, and illicitly for bodybuilding usually are permanent. Androgenic changes usually are caused by medications. However, they also can be caused by ovarian tumors and other disorders within the endocrine system. So, if a singer starts to lose high notes and gain better low notes, medical evaluation should be sought to determine the reason and to rule out tumor-induced androgen production.

There also are many non-sex hormone conditions that can affect the voice. Even mild hypothyroidism (low thyroid) can cause the sensation of a veil over the voice. If a voice becomes muffled, especially if the singer also has noticed fatigue, weight gain, temperature intolerance, brittle hair, and sometimes cognitive changes, thyroid testing should be considered. The condition is not uncommon. An estimated 10% of the American population has hypothyroidism, with the condition having been recognized in only about half of them.

Diabetes is an extremely common endocrine system abnormality. We will not discuss it in detail in this chapter, but it can affect the voice through dry mouth, microvascular changes, neurological changes including partial paralysis of the vocal folds and of nerves elsewhere in the body, hearing loss and other effects. Hormone changes from elsewhere in the endocrine system including the pituitary gland, thymus, pancreas, and other structures also can cause voice changes. Not all physicians are familiar with these problems. So, it is wise for singers to be "informed consumers" and to ask about them when symptoms raise the possibility of a hormone-induced voice change.

47

Don't know about conditions and medicine that tend to make you bleed

Vocal fold hemorrhage, or bleeding into a vocal fold, can be a career-ending event, although that usually is not the outcome. When a singer ruptures a blood vessel in a vocal fold, a hematoma (or blood blister) usually occurs. It is unusual for a singer to cough up blood, although that might be better since it would indicate that the hematoma had been evacuated. If a hematoma occurs on a vocal fold and involves just the upper surface, it might not affect the voice substantially, especially right away. However, the normal mucosal wave courses over the upper surface, not just on the vibratory margin. So, if a hematoma fails to resolve and turns to scar, even on the superior surface that can be problematic. If the hematoma involves the contact margin, sudden voice change is common. Most physicians agree that voice rest (silence) is advisable until the blood in the hematoma resorbs. Once that happens and the mucosa is back in contact with underlying tissues, even if the vocal fold remains discolored and stiff, soft phonation usually is safe, ideally under the supervision of a voice pathologist and a singing voice specialist. However, if a singer continues to "sing through" hoarseness following such a hemorrhage, the repeated trauma may prevent resorption, possibly cause additional bleeding, and potentially lead to scar that causes permanent hoarseness. So, singers should make every effort to avoid hemorrhage; and if they suspect that bleeding has occurred, they should be silent until their vocal folds have been examined (as soon as possible).

In other chapters, we have discussed some conditions that predispose to vocal fold hemorrhage such as the premenstrual hormonal environment. Voice abuse/misuse, particularly loud yelling or singing, can cause vocal fold trauma that leads to blood vessel rupture. However, such problems are particularly likely to occur if singers have ingested medications or other substances that function as "blood thinners" and predispose to bleeding in the vocal folds and elsewhere. There are many such substances. As a micro surgeon, the author (RTS) provides patients preoperatively with a list of medications and other substances that should be avoided before surgery, many of them for 10 to 14 days (especially aspirin products), and usually for a few days after surgery. The list that we distribute to our patients contains 318 substances, and even that is incomplete. So, listing all of them is beyond the scope of this chapter; but they can be found on the Internet. However, some are used quite commonly and are worth emphasis in this chapter. These include aspirin products (often found in cold medicines and labeled as salicylic acid) including aspirin, buffer and Excedrin, among others; Alka-Seltzer, ibuprofen (Motrin, Advil and others), dong quai, echinacea, Flagyl, garlic, ginger, ginkgo, horseradish, licorice, Midol, Naprosyn and other nonsteroidal anti-inflammatory drugs, Pepto-Bismol, Plavix, Sinutab, St. John's Wort, vitamin C, vitamin E and vitamin K (especially vitamin E). These medicines function as anticoagulants. They can be dangerous at any time. However, if they are taken in conjunction with conditions that already predisposed to hemorrhage, the risk is even greater. Such conditions include laryngitis, abdominal pain or cramps that impair support, premenstrual hormonal environment, and others. Unfortunately, these are conditions that are most likely to lead to singers to take such medicines. Instead, they should consult their physicians (ideally their laryngologists) and use safe alternatives.

48

Work to hear yourself

Singers are trained using auditory feedback. That is, we listen to ourselves and make adjustments to the sound based upon what we hear. However, that approach can create problems when we are in environments that make it difficult for us to hear our own voices.

The Lombard effect has been recognized since 1911. It is the tendency to speak more loudly than our baseline in the presence of background noise. In general, voice intensity increases by about 0.38dB for every 1dB increase in noise above 55dB sound pressure level. Normal conversation usually takes place at about 60dB or less. Private businesses without extensive speaking typically have a noise level of about 50–55dB. At about 30 feet, a small truck accelerating produces over 80dB. A commercial jetliner has an ambient noise level of about 92dB. The sound in a loud restaurant typically ranges around 76–80dB; a classical music concert usually is in the 70–90dB range, although the sound within the orchestra can reach 110dB; and church choirs often produce 80–95dB. So, talking during rehearsals can be hazardous. Rock bands may produce 90–120dB, and the drum set alone can account for 105–110dB. So, talking at noisy restaurants, in airplanes, over music, and in similar environments is likely to trigger the Lombard effect. Moreover, 0.38dB per dB of background noise is more than it seems. Decibels or logarithmic. So, for example, if you have a noisy factory machine producing 90dB and turn on a second one producing 90dB, the resultant sound will be noticeably louder, but it will measure only 93dB.

Bars, restaurants, weddings, and similar environments are not the only places in which singers are exposed to substantial background noise. Singing in choirs, with orchestras, and/or rock bands also makes singers compete with background noise; and they often strain to be heard, singing or speaking, more loudly than is safe. Well-trained classical singers are trained to ameliorate this problem by learning to sing using tactile feedback ("by feel") rather than auditory feedback ("by ear"). Rock and pop singers who might not have similar training, and who are competing with much louder instruments in many cases, solve the problem by using monitor speakers or monitor ear inserts that direct sound of the amplified singer's voice to him/her. Failing to use appropriate technique and/or monitor speakers/inserts is likely to lead the singer to sing too loudly and too forcefully in an effort to be heard. This puts the singer at risk of not only hoarseness and voice fatigue, but also of serious voice injury including vocal fold tears, masses and hemorrhages.

This chapter does not include all potentially risky environments, but it should be noted that impaired auditory feedback can occur from conditions other than loud background noise. For example, singing in venues with poor acoustics, and especially singing in an outdoor theater or stadium, can make it very difficult for a singer to hear his/her own voice. Such an environment can lead a singer to work to be heard; and that can result in a serious vocal fold injury.

It is important for singers to be able to monitor their voices, but struggling to do so is hazardous. The solution is mastering techniques and technologies and using them wisely. This can facilitate safe singing in almost any environment.

49

Work too much

We have noted before that singing is an athletic activity. Like other athletic activities, singers require rest in order to perform optimally. Of course, singers also need to pay rent and to eat. It is not unusual for young singers to hold two or three jobs to meet (or almost meet) their financial obligations. Some of the problems associated with working too hard were discussed in chapter 9. Adequate rest, including sleep, is essential for normal function of muscles and nerves, normal lubrication of the vocal folds and other parts of the respiratory tract, maintenance of normal biochemical and metabolic body functions, and for other reasons. Working to the point at which adequate sleep is sacrificed is counterproductive.

However, the physical consequences of working too much are not the only problems. We will not review the consequences of psychological stress on artistic performance. Psychological stress often interferes with sleep, can impair mental health, and has many other consequences, many of which were discussed in chapter 38 of the previous volume in this series. Many of these issues are self-evident to singers. However, there is another factor associated with working too much that is discussed only rarely.

At all stages of a singing career, a singer requires practice, the ability to concentrate and remember what is learned, and the time to learn more about music than just the notes. Singing requires artistry; and artistry requires that the singer "has something to say" regardless of how beautifully the notes are sung. That is one of the important factors that separates singing from the playing of musical instruments. As an example, one of us (RTS) remembers well a rehearsal of Othello during which a singer sang all the notes correctly and with beautiful voice, but with no sense of the drama. The director interrupted her to ask about her interpretation of the part. It came out that she had heard of Shakespeare but had never read any (although she was an advanced professional singer with a graduate degree in voice), and she not only had never read Othello, but she also did not realize that it was a play that had been written by Shakespeare. Such lack of artistic depth does not lead to great singing. If all we want its beautiful notes, we can get them from a cello or a French horn (sometimes). As singers, we need to know more of literature, life, love, hate, death and other components of the world than just the words and notes on the page. Becoming an educated person requires time not only to learn but also to reflect. This is true not only for classical singers singing opera. Musical theater, pop and jazz singers who are successful know a great deal about life and sing from the heart. Most of them did not learn it working 18 hours a day.

We recognize that there are many pressures on the singers, and that they have to do what it takes to survive. However, singers also should consider that NOT taking that third job might be yet another reasonable sacrifice for their career. Working too much compromises the body, the mind and the art.

50

Don't be your own advocate

It is extremely important for singers to be informed consumers and knowledgeable advocates for themselves. This is true for voice care more than it is for many other areas of medicine. The first modern paper teaching doctors how to take care of singers was not published until 1981[1] ; the first ear, nose and throat textbook with a chapter on care of the professional voice was not published until 1986 [2] ; and the first book on care of the professional voice appeared in 1991.[3] Formal fellowship programs to teach ear, nose and throat doctors the subspecialty of laryngology/care the professional voice also started relatively recently. Even in the United States, which has more training programs than most other countries, there are only about 30 fellowship programs for the more than 300 otolaryngologists who graduate from residency each year; and many of those fellowship programs do not emphasize professional voice care. All should cover the topic to some extent, but many focus on swallowing disorders, airway disorders or neurolaryngology which also are components of the field. That means that there are a great many excellent ear, nose and throat doctors in practice who know relatively little about the current state of the art in voice care, and there are even more who have no expertise in caring for singers. For that reason, it is essential for singers to know enough to be able to judge whether they are being cared for by a voice expert, and whether the advice that they are receiving makes sense. For example, a singer who is told that they have "vocal nodules" and require immediate surgery should know several things in order to put that device in perspective. First, unless the singer has been evaluated by high-quality strobovideolaryngoscopy, it usually is not possible to differentiate a nodule from other benign masses such as cysts and polyps. If the examination has been performed only under continuous light (even if a scope has been placed through the nose), the diagnosis should be considered uncertain. Second, although "nodules" are relatively uncommon in adults (as compared with cysts and other lesions), when nodules occur, approximately 90% resolve or become asymptomatic with excellent voice therapy alone. Surgery usually is not required; and urgent surgery for nodules is never required. Urgent surgery for benign vocal fold masses usually is indicated only if they obstruct or threaten to obstruct the airway, and that virtually never happens with nodules. Other misdiagnoses and incorrect treatment recommendations are fairly common and may be made by excellent doctors who simply never received specialized training in voice care; and they might not even know that there is a great deal of information that they don't know, even though they are superb at managing other ear, nose and throat problems.

Consequently, singers need to know enough to know when to follow advice, and when to say "thank you" and go find another opinion. Good physicians are always anxious to help their patients and often think of ways to try to do so, not realizing that their lack of special expertise may lead them to make counterproductive suggestions. If singers are not certain that they are under the care of an otolaryngologist with real expertise in caring for singers, they should not be shy about seeking other opinions before agreeing to care, especially in nonemergent circumstances.

References

1. Sataloff RT. Professional Singers: The Science and Art of Clinical Care. *American Journal of Otolaryngology*. 1981;2(3):251–266.

2. Sataloff, R.T. The Professional Voice. In: Cummings, C.W., Frederickson, J.M., Harker, L.A., Krause, C.J., Schuller, D.E. (Eds) *Otolaryngology-Head and Neck Surgery*. St. Louis, MO: C.V. Mosby; 1986:2029–2056.

3. Sataloff, R.T. *Professional Voice: The Science and Art of Clinical Care*. New York, NY: Raven Press;1991.

Author Biographies

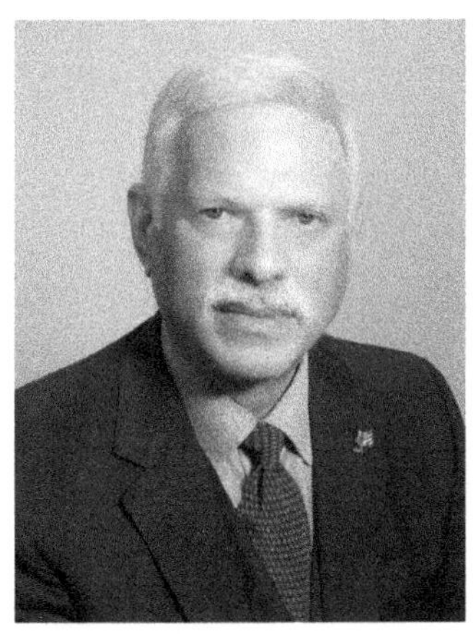

Robert T. Sataloff, M.D., D.M.A., F.A.C.S. is Professor and Chair, Department of Otolaryngology-Head and Neck Surgery and Senior Associate Dean for Clinical Academic Specialties, Drexel University College of Medicine. Dr. Sataloff is Director of Otolaryngology Education at Lankenau Medical Center. He also holds Adjunct Professorships in the Departments of Otolaryngology – Head and Neck Surgery at Thomas Jefferson University and the Philadelphia College of Osteopathic Medicine; and he is on the faculty of the Academy of Vocal Arts. He serves as Conductor of the Thomas Jefferson University Choir.

Dr. Sataloff is also a professional singer and singing teacher. He holds an undergraduate degree from Haverford College in Music Theory and Composition; graduated from Jefferson Medical College, Thomas Jefferson University; received a Doctor of Musical Arts in Voice Performance from Combs College of Music; and he completed Residency in Otolaryngology – Head and Neck Surgery and a Fellowship in Otology, Neurotology and Skull Base Surgery at the University of Michigan.

Dr. Sataloff is Chair of the Boards of Directors of the Voice Foundation and of the American Institute for Voice and Ear Research. He also has served as Chair of the Board of Governors of Graduate Hospital; President of the American Laryngological Association, the International Association of Phonosurgery, the Pennsylvania Academy of Otolaryngology – Head and Neck Surgery, and The American Society of Geriatric Otolaryngology, and in numerous other leadership positions. Dr. Sataloff is Editor-in-Chief of the *Journal of Voice*; Editor Emeritus of *Ear, Nose and Throat Journal*; Associate Editor of the *Journal of Singing*; on the Editorial Board of *Medical Problems of Performing Artists* and is an editorial reviewer for numerous otolaryngology journals. He has written over 1,000 publications including 77 books, and he has been awarded more than $5 million in research funding. His H-index is 47 (as of April 2024). He has invented more than 75 laryngeal microsurgical instruments distributed currently by Integra Medical, ossicular replacement prostheses produced by Grace Medical, and a novel laryngeal prosthesis (patent pending). He holds a patent on a unique thyroplasty implant. His medical practice is limited to care of the professional voice and to otology/neurotology/skull base surgery. Dr. Sataloff has developed numerous novel surgical procedures including total temporal bone resection for formerly untreatable skull base malignancy, laryngeal microflap and mini-microflap procedures, vocal fold lipoinjection, vocal fold lipoimplantation, and others. Dr. Sataloff is recognized as one of the founders of the field of voice, having written the first modern comprehensive article on care of singers, and the first chapter and book on care of the professional voice, as well as having influenced the evolution of the field through his own efforts and through the Voice Foundation for over 4 decades. Dr. Sataloff has been recognized by Best Doctors in America (Woodward White Athens) every year since 1992, Philadelphia Magazine since 1997, and Castle Connolly's "America's Top Doctors" since 2002.

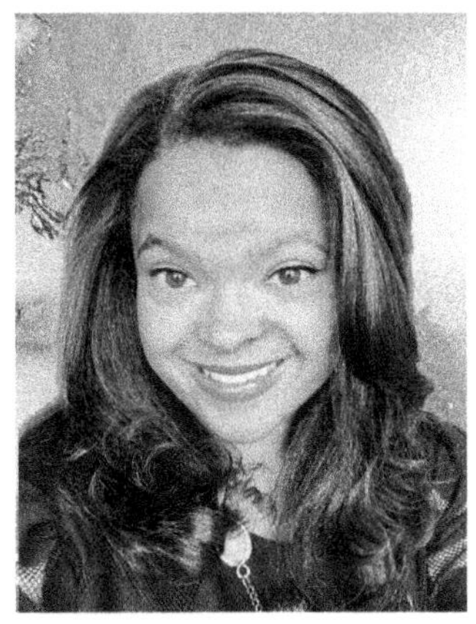

Christina L. Mancheni, D.M.A. is an Assistant Professor of Voice in the Department of Music at Boise State University in Boise, Idaho. Dr. Mancheni is a professional singer who has performed on the operatic stage and has appeared often as a concert, recital, and chamber soloist. She is also an avid performer of various other styles of music including operetta, musical theater, and contemporary commercial music.

She has performed for several companies and festivals both nationally and internationally in addition to winning numerous awards and competitions. She holds an undergraduate degree in Voice Performance and Doctor of Musical Arts in Voice Performance from the University of Nevada, Las Vegas; and she received a Master of Music in Voice Performance from Miami University of Ohio. Dr. Mancheni has presented master classes, clinics, and recitals regionally. She is also an active member of the Voice Foundation and the National Association of Teachers Singing (NATS) where she has adjudicated regional competitions.

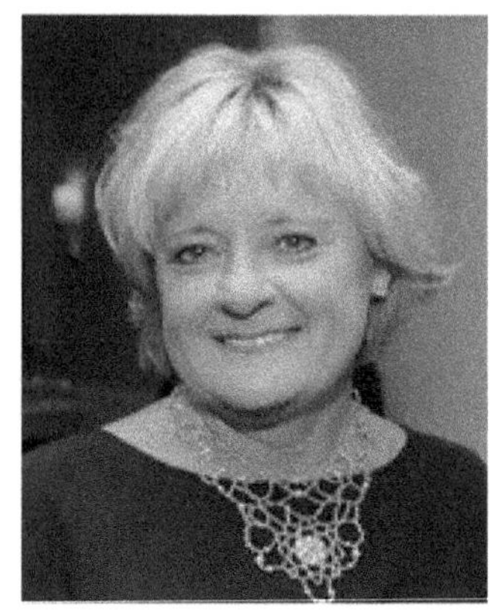

Mary J. Hawkshaw, B.S.N., R.N., CORLN is Research Professor and Vice Chair for Academic Initiatives in the Department of Otolaryngology – Head and Neck Surgery at Drexel University College of Medicine. She has been associated with Dr. Robert Sataloff, Philadelphia Ear, Nose & Throat Associates and the American Institute for Voice & Ear Research (AIVER) since 1986.

Ms. Hawkshaw graduated from Shadyside Hospital School of Nursing in Pittsburgh and received a Bachelor of Science degree in Nursing from Thomas Jefferson University in Philadelphia. In addition to her specialized clinical activities, she has been involved extensively in research and teaching. She mentors medical students, residents, and laryngology fellows, and has been involved in teaching research, writing and editing for over three decades. In collaboration with Dr. Sataloff, she has co-authored 185 articles, 108 book chapters, and 20 textbooks. She is on the Editorial Boards of the Journal of Voice and Ear, Nose and Throat Journal. She has served as Secretary/Treasurer of AIVER since 1988 and was named Executive Director of AIVER in January 2000. She has served on the Board of Directors of the Voice Foundation since 1990. Ms. Hawkshaw has been an active member of the Society of Otorhinolaryngology and Head-Neck Nurses since 1998. She is recognized nationally and internationally for her extensive contributions to care of the professional voice.

www.ingramcontent.com/pod-product-compliance
Lightning Source LLC
La Vergne TN
LVHW021140160826
845679LV00023B/1987

* 9 7 8 1 9 0 9 0 8 2 7 5 5 *